# Diabetes: An Everyday Guide

# Diabetes:
# An Everyday Guide

Sasha Fenton

ZAMBEZI PUBLISHING LTD

Published in 2008 by
Zambezi Publishing Ltd
P.O. Box 221 Plymouth, Devon PL2 2YJ (UK)
web: www.zampub.com  email: info@zampub.com

Copyright © 2008 Sasha Fenton
Cover design: © 2008 Jan Budkowski
Sasha Fenton has asserted her moral right
to be identified as the author of this work in terms of
the Copyright, Designs and Patents Act 1988

British Library Cataloguing-in-Publication Data:
A catalogue record for this book is available from
the British Library

Typeset by Zambezi Publishing Ltd, Plymouth UK
Printed and bound in the UK by Lightning Source (UK) Ltd

*(ISBN-13)*:  978-1-903065-68-6

135798642

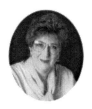

## *About the Author*

Sasha is the author of over 120 books on Mind, Body and Spirit subjects, and she has broadcast and lectured all over the world for the past 30 years. However, Sasha says that the research for this book took far longer than it normally takes to write half a dozen of her usual style of book!

Not only does Sasha come from a family of diabetics, but she lost her first husband and two good friends to ailments directly caused, or complicated by diabetes, and she has had her own problems with pre-diabetes and diet-controlled diabetes for many years.

Sasha lives in Devon with her husband, Jan Budkowski and their much-loved dog, Pippa. Sasha has two children and two granddaughters. So, far, they are all healthy and Sasha hopes they will stay that way.

## *Acknowledgments*

With grateful thanks to Sue Pearson, who asked me to write this book, to Yvonne Aitken, for her encouragement and for checking the medical information, and to Dr. S. Hobbs for his unfailing guidance and advice.

To Jan, who checked my findings, did a lot of the research and edited this book.

# Contents

*Prologue with Porridge*     3

1  *Diagnosis Diabetes*     5

2  *About Diabetes*     13

3  *Diets and Diabetes*     21

4  *Frequently Asked Questions*     25

5  *Shock and Stress*     29

6  *Types of Diabetes*     31

7  *My Story*     35

8  *Symptoms*     39

9  *Measurements and Spikes*     45

10  *Diabetes and Sugars*     57

11  *Diabetes and Fats*     63

12  *The Techie Stuff*     69

13  *Other Health Situations*     75

14  *Are You Overweight?*     79

15  *Children*     87

16  *Medicines and Medical People*     91

17  *Being Active*     95

18  *Breakfast*     99

19  *Main Meals*     103

20  *Packed Lunches and Picnics*     109

21  *Desperate Measures*     113

22  *Dining Out and Takeaways*     117

23  *Carbohydrates and Starches*     125

24  *Pulses*     131

25  Proteins                                135

26  Fruit and Vegetables                    139

27  Drinks                                   141

28  Body Care                                149

29  Oh, God, It's Christmas!                 157

30  Travel and Holidays                      161

31  Helpful Ideas                            171

32  Supplements and Natural Remedies         179

    Conclusion                               185

    Bibliography                             187

    Index                                    195

# Prologue with Porridge

*Sue*

Nurse Sue Pearson had taken some blood from my arm, and she was writing the details on the vial when we started to chat. It turned out that Sue has pre-diabetes herself, and she is staving off full-blown type 2 diabetes by eating carefully and taking some exercise. We both laughed at our fondness for porridge, which we discovered fills us up and doesn't make our blood sugar rise too quickly. Sue is aware that I know a lot about diabetes, but it was what she said next that made me gasp, because she asked me to write a book about it! In all my years of writing, I have never had a book commissioned at my doctor's surgery!

Sue said that she and her colleagues needed a simple, easy-to-read book, to recommend to newly diagnosed type 2 diabetics and for those who struggle to understand how to take care of themselves or of their diabetic loved ones. She told me that patients don't understand that cutting down on cakes just isn't enough, and she also said that it's hard to get the average overweight middle-aged person to understand that some kind of exercise is vital. She told me that many of her patients roundly rejected the idea of doing anything, including something as mild as a daily walk round the block.

### *Yvonne*

Sister Yvonne Aitken lent me books and pointed me in the direction of other material, and she encouraged me all along the way. In time, she checked the draft manuscript for safety and for medical content. Yvonne's ambition is to specialise as a diabetes nurse, and Jan and I wish her every success in her objective.

### *This Book*

I have not gone deeply into the technicalities of medicines, insulin and blood testing regimes, but I have listed other books and many sources of information at the back of this book.

If you are looking into diabetes for the first time, or if your condition isn't too severe, my book will probably give you enough information for daily life, but you will need more technical information about specific drugs, treatments and monitoring, so check out the information section at the back of this book and join "Diabetes UK". (See the back of this book for details.)

The one major factor that arose from every single source that I looked into, is that diabetes responds very well to self-help. Above all, it means keeping blood glucose (blood sugar) levels within the correct limits, along with paying attention to the areas of the body that are most vulnerable to damage. A very important point that is missed by many people, including some in the medical world, is that every diabetic is an individual and each one of us responds differently. We each have to find out what makes our blood glucose rise and what keeps us on an even keel.

# 1

# Diagnosis Diabetes

*What Is Diabetes? ~ Who's this Book for? ~ Shock of Diagnosis ~ The Good News ~ Other People ~ Allow Yourself to Mourn ~ Some Odds and Ends*

*There are a lot of people in this world who spend so much time watching their health that they haven't the time to enjoy it.*
Josh Billings

In this book, I try to reach two objectives - the first being to tell you about this perplexing condition, and the second being to show you how taking control of your lifestyle can save you a great deal of aggravation. Did you know that:

~ In the western world, the major causes of blindness and limb amputation are due to diabetes?

~ There are over 2 million diabetics in the UK, with about 750,000 more undiagnosed (24 million diabetics in the USA, or 8 per cent of the population)?

~ Obesity is one of the key factors in developing this affliction?

~ Latest research has found that in the UK, more than 26,000 people die annually due to diabetic complications? This is twice as many as the 12,500 UK women who die each year from breast cancer.

You can check such research data, and much more, on the Diabetes UK website (www.diabetes.org.uk).

Small changes, such as switching from "full fat" soft drinks to the sugar-free variety, and taking up salsa dancing or gardening in preference to dozing life away on the sofa, can deflect disaster. No other chronic ailment requires as much knowledge as diabetes, and none respond to self-help as successfully. In some cases, type 2 diabetes can be kept away for several years (or even forever) by a few simple adaptations to your lifestyle.

What I *don't* go into here is passive experience of being a patient. I don't describe visits to a clinic or describe the various tests and treatments that you might be given. Neither do I go into the difficulties faced by parents of diabetic children. I will cover some (and perhaps all) of those things in a follow-up book, but in the meantime, *this* book seeks to put knowledge and power in *your* hands and to save you from as much grief, pain, stress and loss as possible. If you are the relative of a diabetic, this book will help you to understand this bewildering ailment and show what you can do to help.

## *What is Diabetes?*

We all consume food and drink and process it inside the body; then the body takes what it needs in the form of proteins, vitamins and so on, and tosses out what it doesn't need. In some cases, the body stores material that it thinks might need later - the most obvious example of this being fat. When we diet and exercise, we dig into the fat store and reduce it - for a while, at least. Where diabetes is concerned, the body can't process sugars and carbohydrates the way that it should. A normal person consumes foodstuffs that convert to glucose for energy, and then stores the glucose in the liver until it's needed. If the normal person then plays a game of football or boogies the night away, this stored glucose is sent to the organs and muscles where it gives them some much-needed extra oomph. Even when a normal person doesn't exercise, the body releases insulin and converts the glucose to something useful, or destroys what it doesn't need.

This is the difference between diabetic folk and the rest of the world. If a non-diabetic ate a meal of pizza with garlic bread, followed by dessert, accompanied by a sugary soft drink and finished off with sugared coffee and a super-sweet liqueur, his blood glucose level would rise. A couple of hours later, however, the normal person's blood glucose level would have dropped back down again. In the case of a diabetic, the level rises and then stays up, lingering in the body and doing all kinds of harm.

We don't have enough insulin to bring the overload of blood glucose down, and our livers and kidneys are not great at processing the insulin that we *do* make. This lingering blood glucose then goes to work, destroying many parts of our bodies. The good news is that the destruction wrought by diabetes doesn't happen overnight, and it can be controlled. With a bit of care, a diabetic should live a normal life and do everything that non-diabetics do. Some very special, very serious cases may not live a long life, but the vast majority of us do, as long as we take care of ourselves.

*

It's worth reading this book through once, to get a grasp of the condition as a whole, but I suggest that you then keep it on a convenient shelf for reference. For instance, you might want to check the holiday section before jetting off, or you may wish to look at the list of symptoms when you happen to feel off colour, or when something strange happens to your body. You may need to check certain foodstuffs or take advice before going out for a special meal.

## *Who is This Book For?*

This book is for those who have been recently diagnosed or those who find themselves living or working closely with a diabetic. It is particularly suitable if:

~ You've recently been diagnosed.
~ You've been told that you're in danger of getting diabetes.
~ You come from a family of diabetics.

~  You're a relative, carer, friend or colleague of a diabetic.
~  You worry that your children might get diabetes.

### *Shock of Diagnosis*

Even if you suspect that you have diabetes, it still comes as a shock when you are formally diagnosed. Before you descend into depression or feel that your life is over, bear in mind that this ailment can be controlled, and that is more than can be said for many other ailments. Once you get a grip, eat better food, get some exercise and take medication (if needs be) you will feel a lot better.

Diabetes is a very confusing ailment. Its causes are confusing and its management is even more confusing. Dietary ideas that held sway for previous generations are now considered old hat, but there's still a lot of disagreement about dietary management for diabetics. The latest ideas are based on keeping your weight down and limiting the consumption of harmful sugars, carbohydrates, fats and salt.

### *The Good News*

Most of the time you don't look ill, so you won't get much sympathy. The upside is that your appearance won't prejudice employers against you. The vast majority of jobs are unaffected by diabetes, so there may be no need for you to tell your boss or anyone at your workplace about it. On the other hand, if you have a trusted friend or colleague at work, it's worth letting them know what they must do for you if you become ill.

The second good thing is that diabetes can be controlled, and much of this is in your own hands. A third benefit only comes into view over time. The focus on eating well, being active, looking after yourself and taking a positive attitude to your condition means that in the long term, you will be fitter, livelier, sexier and longer-lived than many of your pals.

### Other People

For most people, diabetes is just a word, and they don't have a clue as to what the diabetes is, or how dangerous it can be if it's neglected. However, when a diabetic is diagnosed, bossy relatives can suddenly appoint themselves as experts who control every bite of food that the poor diabetic takes, and even take charge of home blood testing sessions.

Unfortunately, there are a few arrogant people working in the health field who also have little idea about this ailment, but it doesn't stop them from considering themselves experts, taking every opportunity to boss people around. Here is a true story about a man who had an accident that was unrelated to his diabetes, but that landed him in his local A&E.

When he told the Sister in charge that he was an insulin dependent type 2 diabetic, she snorted and said that there was no such thing and that he really didn't need his insulin. He put his foot down and insisted that she phone the diabetes clinic. When they told her that there were many insulin dependent type 2 diabetics around and that she must allow the poor man to inject his insulin in peace, she complained loudly, "Well, nobody told me about that!"

If you are faced with ignorance and arrogance on this scale, send someone out for a copy of my book and tell them to read it! It will be the least expensive and most effective way of getting them off your back. If this sounds as though I am trying to sell more copies of this book, that's absolutely true, because the more people who read it, the safer and happier we will all become. After the draconian discounts that publishers have to give bookshops and distributors, the money I am likely to make from sales of a successful non-fiction book would probably be enough for me to buy a new pair of shoes. Or if it does really well, two new pairs of shoes!

### Allow Yourself to Mourn

If you feel sad, depressed and fed up at the thought of being on a permanent diet and exercise regime, do yourself a favour and have a good cry. Maybe join an Internet chat room for diabetics, so that you can talk to others who know what you're going through. You're entitled to your feelings and no amount of exhortation to pull yourself together or reminders that there are others far worse off will help. Other people have their problems, but you have yours, and you're perfectly entitled to feel cheesed off about it.

### *Some Odds and Ends...*

Here is a statement from Diabetes UK:

*"Government targets for improving diabetes care may be missed, as local health providers are failing to offer key services".*

The NHS is struggling, so it's more important than ever for you to find out as much as you can about diabetes and how to manage and treat it. Look after yourself so you don't have to push NHS workers into looking after you before it's absolutely necessary. If you need specialist help, ask for it; don't be fobbed off. You may hate to "bother" your doctor, but it isn't the doctor who will become sick, blind and disabled, it's you.

Having said that, our healthcare for diabetic patients is better than that of most other countries.

\*

Health clinic screening for various things often misses the possibility of raised blood glucose, so if you or a family member suspect that they have the problem, ask for a blood test at the clinic or at a pharmacy, because a pharmacist can do this on the spot and the results are available in a minute or two. Just avoid times when the shop is busy. If you know you are pre-diabetic, treat yourself to a blood-testing machine from the pharmacy, so that you can check your own blood glucose once in a while.

\*

A shortage of vitamin D can lead to diabetes, especially type 1 in children and young people. If there is any history of diabetes in your family at all, it's worth asking your doctor about giving your children a suitable vitamin D supplement. Vitamin D is found in milk and it is put into some commercially made bread, but it is mainly found in sunlight. There is no need to put your children or yourself in danger of skin cancer by lying about in the sun, because even a little fresh air and sunlight will help. Pollution in city centres filters sunlight, and our habit of driving kids to and from school cuts down the amount of vitamin D they have access to, so city children and those who don't walk about outside very much may need supplements.

# 2

# About Diabetes

*Diabetes Affects Everything ~ How Dangerous is Diabetes? ~ a Weighty Matter ~ Does it Affect more of One Sex than Another? ~ Ethnicity ~ Causes ~ Not just Humans! ~ Why Me, Why This, Why Now? ~ Checklist*

*Every patient carries his or her own doctor inside.*
Albert Schweitzer

## *Diabetes Affects Everything*

As Sister Yvonne Aitken says, diabetes affects every part of the body and every activity and area of life in ways that other ailments rarely do. Of course, there are unusually severe ailments - say for instance, of the kind that Stephen Hawking has -that affect everything and everybody concerning the sick person. Diabetes doesn't look much from the outside, because a diabetic goes to work, attends social events, plays sports, looks after a family and lives an apparently normal life. But it's not normal. Everything we eat, every place that we visit and every activity that we take up, needs thought and preparation. We must avoid damage and stress to our bodies. We need to accommodate our need for regular medication, regular intake of suitable food, the shoes we choose to wear when playing sports or activities, and we even need to take good account of the temperature and weather.

Diabetes occurs when beta cells in the pancreas no longer do what they were made for, which is to produce enough of the hormone insulin.

In type 1 diabetes, beta cells stop working, so that little or no insulin is produced at all.

In type 2 diabetes, the beta cells produce some insulin, but not enough. The liver may be sluggish and unwilling to process, store and then release insulin into the bloodstream as it should. There may also be weakness in other parts of the body that contributes to the situation.

The muscles and organs of the body need glucose to produce energy and they rely on insulin to push glucose into their cells. When the muscles and organs are starved of glucose, they can't do their job properly, which is why diabetics feel so tired. The problem isn't a shortage of glucose in the body, there's plenty of it, but it sticks in the wrong place, mainly in the blood, liver and kidneys, where it piles up and causes damage. Insulin and other factors enable the movement of glucose from these storehouses into the muscles and other areas where it is needed, and help its conversion into energy. If insulin can't get where it needs to be, if there isn't enough of it being manufactured, or if the body doesn't absorb it well enough, the person becomes diabetic.

## How Dangerous is Diabetes?

Diabetes can have a strange effect on many parts of the body. For instance, the majority of amputations of toes, feet and legs that became gangrenous are due to diabetes, and it's probably one of the main reasons for blindness. It leads to high blood pressure, hardening of the arteries, heart attacks, strokes, kidney dialysis, crumbling bones in the feet and a host of other ailments. It weakens the workings of many parts of the body, so that almost anything can malfunction. Even diabetics who are not badly afflicted suffer some problems, and most get tired easily.

We all know that we should eat properly, exercise several times a week and keep our weight down, and many of us say that that we'll do it when we can get round to it. While this attitude may cause a problem in the long term for a healthy person, it will cause lots of problems in no time at all for a diabetic one! If you have recently been diagnosed with diabetes, you really don't have a choice in the matter. If you keep the disease under control, you can live a normal life. With type 2 diabetes, good control will mean that you may be able to ease back on the amount of medication that you take. Many diabetics can control the disease by diet and exercise alone for a long time. You will need to monitor your condition with occasional blood tests at your surgery and have an annual eye test.

### *A Weighty Matter*

Not everyone with type 2 diabetes is overweight but many sufferers are, and that doesn't help the situation. The bad news is that type 2 diabetes actually makes a body hang on to unnecessary weight. Worse still, it makes the sufferer hungry, and even when a diabetic doesn't feel hungry, he or she mustn't skip meals. Worse still, some medicines pile on the pounds. One person I know looked normal before he was diagnosed, and now that he is taking pills, he looks like the Michelin man!

Our society tolerates things that other societies don't, but conversely it doesn't tolerate some things that others do. For example, in some countries, if a woman spends a moment or two discussing an incorrectly delivered letter with the postman, she is liable to be beaten for talking to a man that isn't her husband. In our society, talking to the postman is fine, but being overweight is sinful. Thin people are considered more valuable and worthy members of society than fat ones. Can you imagine a very fat person trying to become our Prime Minister or President of the USA?

### *Does it Affect More of One Sex than Another?*

I always saw diabetes as a mainly male disease, and indeed, it once was. Within my own family, the diabetics are (or were) my great grandfather, grandfather and four male cousins. I am the only diabetic woman. Nowadays, statistics show that diabetes is fairly evenly spread across the sexes, although it seems that more women are going down with diabetes nowadays, possibly due to poor diet and lifestyle. Women sometimes become diabetic during pregnancy and they recover after the birth.

### Ethnicity

Every book I've come across states that diabetes is more prevalent in Afro-Caribbean and South East Asian communities than in other races. None of the books or pamphlets that I read mention Jewish people, but it is common among Jews and I have even heard it called "the Jewish disease".

> **Type 1 diabetes requires insulin injections. It can't easily be controlled, but its worst effects can be minimised by all-round healthy living. The good news is that type 1 diabetics are usually slim.**

### Causes

It is said that those whose ancestors went short of food have an inbuilt ability to hoard sugars in the body. In the UK, the shortages of food in the First World War, the depression of the 1930s, the rationing during the Second World War and the worse rationing that we put up with after the war ended, meant that the parents of the "war babies" and "baby-boomers" didn't get enough to eat. In theory, wartime rationing was designed to give everyone his or her basic needs, but sometimes greedy and selfish personalities took more than their fair share, leaving others to starve. Many people throughout Europe starved during the Second World War, and population movement means that the descendants of these people now live all around Western Europe, the USA and the British Commonwealth.

Another factor is that type 2 diabetes has always been associated with old age, and we live longer than previous generations did, so that also makes us vulnerable. Older people are less active and they may not pay proper attention to their food intake.

There have always been a few people who were uncommonly fat, but nowadays, one look around any provincial high street shows many fat people wobbling around the shops. Perhaps part of the reason for this is the end of the traditional family, where someone cooked proper meals. I have single friends who live exclusively on pizza and takeaways, while others can cook, but they are too busy with the sofa, television, their fags and "puff" to bother making a nice casserole. People like me spend our lives chained to a typing chair and a computer. We get tired from our work and then we don't have much energy left for sport or activities.

### Not Just Humans!

Unbelievably, diabetes can also be a problem for dogs, and probably for other pets as well! Many people feed their dogs leftovers, and if the food that we eat is unhealthy, it won't do the dog much good, either!

### Why Me, Why This, Why Now?

Diabetes isn't a punishment from God, and neither is caring for a diabetic child a punishment from God. Life may be hard, but it isn't because you did something bad. If you believe in karma, you will know that the theory states that you will experience all kinds of circumstances during many lifetimes, so the lesson for this lifetime is to cope with diabetes in yourself or to care for a child who has diabetes.

If you don't like this kind of spiritual philosophy, try this bit of homespun wisdom from my late Grandma: "Everyone has their share of aggravation in life. It may come when you're young or when you're old, and it may come in one shape or in another, but it will come."

**Try this Checklist:**

A   Do you only feel thirsty after several hours without having a drink?
B   Do you feel thirsty all the time?

A   Is your weight stable?
B   Are you losing weight very rapidly recently without dieting?
C   Have you gained weight recently without doing anything different?

A   Do you normally have fresh breath?
B   Do you often have a dry mouth and bad breath?
C   Does your breath ever smell like nail polish or pear drops?

A   Do you sleep through the night?
B   Do you get up to use the loo during the night?

A   Do you sleep well and wake up refreshed?
B   Do you wake up feeling like death warmed up?

A   Do you potter about when you get up in the morning?
B   Do you rush to the loo, swig a glass of water and then put the kettle on?

A   Does your skin just get dry in particularly hot or cold weather?
B   Is you skin, dry, sore and peculiar; and is it bothering you?

A   Do cuts heal quickly?
B   Do cuts and scrapes take a donkey's age to heal?

A   Is your eyesight reliable?
B   Are your eyes clear at times and blurry at other times?

A   Do your hands and feet rarely, if ever, tingle?
B   Do you get tingling feelings on most days and nights?

A    Are you generally well?
B    Do you often get thrush, cystitis and tummy bugs?

A    Do you bounce back from colds?
B    Do you dread colds?

A    Are your teeth reasonably good?
B    Are your teeth and gums prone to abscesses?

A    Do you feel even the slightest discomfort?
B    Do you have a high tolerance to pain?

**"A" answers suggest that you probably don't have diabetes**
**"B" answers suggest that you probably do have it**
**"C" answers also suggest that you may have diabetes**

# 3

# Diets and Diabetes

---

*Is there a Special Diet? ~ Ordinary Food is Fine ~ Information and Resources ~ Other Information ~ Vegan Evangelism ~ Common Sense*

*"No but, yes but, no but, yes but..."*
As said by Vicki in Little Britain.

### Is there Such Thing as a Diabetic Diet?
Well, no, there isn't such a thing, but in a way there *is*. Confusion rules OK!

### Ordinary Food is Fine
There's no need to buy quinoa seeds, buckwheat, goji beans, brown rice or any product that looks and tastes like hamster droppings, because normal food, such as meat, potatoes and vegetables, fish, salads or a vegetarian diet are absolutely fine. The biggest snag concerns those things that rapidly turn to glucose within the body, so we are talking about sweets, cakes, biscuits, buns, white bread, chocolate, sugary sweet drinks and desserts. You will need to cut back on things that contain white flour and possibly things that contain cornstarch if they happen to make your diabetes worse. The second main problem is saturated fat, excess fats and fatty junk food. A third problem is salt.

Once you get the balance right, you can afford the occasional treat, such as eating a piece of someone's birthday cake, or a Chinese takeaway, but you mustn't slither back into bad habits on a permanent basis. The old idea that you can't eat any sugar whatsoever and that you must severely restrict carbohydrates (starchy foods) has now gone, so you shouldn't feel hungry all the time. The bad news is that you just can't gobble down a 500g bar of Cadbury's fruit and nut when you feel the urge.

You may be able to adapt favourite recipes by substituting sweeteners, fruit sugar, fruit or fruit juice, lower calorie spreads, good oils and healthier choices. You will have to experiment a bit. There are plenty of things you *can* eat, and I've listed lots of cookery books in the resources chapter at the back of this book. Every diabetic is different, so you will need to study yourself and develop your own eating regime. If you decide to go on a diet, you must eat regularly and not skip meals.

**Make milk puddings, such as rice, tapioca and semolina with semi-skimmed milk and Splenda. It tastes just as good as the cream and sugar version, and the calorie, cholesterol and glucose content are dramatically lower. Canderel releases damaging chemicals when heated up; it also loses its sweetness, so only add Canderel powder to cooked food.**

## Information

You will find a list of books about diabetes, and specialised cook books at the end of this book. There's a torrent of information on the Internet, although much of it is American, making their measurements and recipes hard for us in the UK to understand. If you're a type 1 diabetic, you will get medical help and advice from your surgery. Type 2 diabetics may get help or they may be given a leaflet and then left to get on with things. There are also books (and Internet information) on the market for those with heart problems, high blood pressure and high cholesterol.

*Vegan Evangelism*

There's one book that I've come across during my researches that has an air of hysterical evangelism about it. The author believes that he has found the key to the Holy Grail, the roadmap to health and so on. The author and his colleagues show how they have experimented with absolute veganism, and discovered that it has a beneficial effect on cholesterol. This isn't surprising, because all cholesterol bearing items, such as meat, poultry, fish, shellfish, eggs, cheese, butter and milk are off the menu. Even milk is replaced by liquid made from soya or almonds. The book advocates restricting all fats and oils, including vegetable oil. Needless to say, the patient is exhorted to eat lots of brown rice and brown pasta. Apparently, apart from lowering cholesterol levels, this has a positive effect on diabetes and a beneficial effect on arthritis.

If you happen to be a vegan, this regime may suit you very well, but for the rest of us, it's too strange and too difficult to live with, especially if we have to feed a family and eat out from time to time. I also worry about the high number of recipes with soya and mushrooms in, as that can cause candida in the gut. All in all, I tend to be sceptical about extremes of any kind.

Coincidentally, it has recently been mentioned in the news that someone has suffered brain damage from a lack of sodium, due to one of those extreme diets that help you lose weight swiftly. Consult your dietician or diabetes nurse before doing anything extreme.

*Common Sense*

The best diet is something that keeps your blood glucose down, and if it also helps you to lose weight that's a bonus, but that needn't be an aim in itself - it's the blood glucose level that matters. Everybody is different. For instance, I know that if I eat more than a small amount of food products containing white flour, my blood glucose goes up quickly and then stays up. The answer is - as the old saying goes - "Know thyself!"

# 4

# Frequently Asked Questions

---

*Can you Continue Working? ~ Famous Diabetics ~ Not only Diabetics Benefit ~ Will your Children Develop Diabetes? ~ Bling and ID cards ~ Help with Costs*

*"I told you I was ill!"*
Spike Milligan was a hypochondriac, so he had this message engraved on his gravestone.

### Can You Continue working?

Like so much about this ailment, the answer isn't totally cut and dried. It shouldn't stop you from working in the vast majority of jobs, but diabetes is unacceptable in some careers because you could place your life or the lives of others in danger. The questionable jobs are those in transport, being in charge of passengers, the armed forces and some forms of police work, jobs that involve climbing pylons or scaffolding, plus mining and diving. You can take part in most sports and activities, although some extreme or endurance sports will require special steps.

Interestingly, there was a story in the news only recently about a lorry driver who lost consciousness and ploughed into a couple who were out for a walk, killing the woman and crippling the man. The man hadn't looked after himself and he hadn't had a blood test for a year! He had become very hypoglycaemic, which made him behave as though he was extremely drunk. The judge said that the lorry driver should have taken proper responsibility for his condition, and sentenced him to four years imprisonment. The driver said that he wished that *he* had died, rather than being responsible for death and injury to others. The sad thing is that this situation was entirely preventable.

If you are on medication or insulin, you will need to inform the DVLA and your motor insurers. You will certainly need to put the information on any holiday insurance form. It is also wise to wear the likes of a MedicAlert bracelet or necklace, and to have a note in your wallet or purse about your condition and what first aid you might need in an emergency.

### *Famous Diabetics*

Some famous diabetics include the following:
~ Olympic gold medallist, Steve Redgrave
~ Author of the Inspector Morse books, Colin Dexter
~ The elderly singer and actor, Elaine Stritch
~ Film star, Halle Berry
~ Comedian, Jimmy Tarbuk
~ Film star, Sharon Stone
~ Miss America 1999, Nicole Johnson
~ Singer, Ella Fitzgerald
~ TV personality, Larry King
~ Film star, Elizabeth Taylor
~ Singer, Meat Loaf
~ Composer, Andrew Lloyd Webber
~ Heavy weight boxer, "Smokin' Joe" Frazier
~ Film Star, Mae West
~ Film star, Spencer Tracy
~ The one and only Elvis Presley
~ Singer, Johnny Cash
~ The politician, John Prescott. (This also shows that a diabetic can still live a full sex life!)

### Not only Diabetics Benefit

If you improve your diet, the chances are that you and your family as a whole will eat better. This could have a magical effect on your children, as the reduction in sugars and food additives will improve their concentration and their behaviour.

### Bling and ID Cards

You can buy special bracelets and necklaces from a number of sources, of which the most common is probably the firm mentioned below. These vary in price and type, from inexpensive and basic to fancy and expensive.

You can even have an ordinary bracelet made up and engrave your details on the back of it, but if you do, ensure that the front clearly shows the "caduceus" symbol that will alert medical people anywhere in the world that you have a problem. Look up other sources using an Internet search engine.

MedicAlert
1 Bridge Wharf
156 Caledonian Road
London N1 9UU
www.medicalert.org.uk

> The caduceus symbol belongs to the Roman god, Mercury, or the equivalent Greek god, Hermes. He saw two snakes fighting so he threw his staff down between them, at which point they stopped fighting and slithered off. Mercury was the god of medicine, alchemists, messages, psychology, local travel, termini, trickery and thieves!

Make up a card saying what your condition is, showing the medicines that you take and giving your doctor's name, address and phone number. Keep this in your wallet or purse. If you want us to make up a laminated card, email us or drop us a line. We have to charge for this, as it takes time and materials, but if you can't get it done locally for some reason, we will try to help.

## *Help with Costs*

If you're on prescribed medication in the UK, you can get free blood testing strips. If you're diet controlled, you may have to pay for everything, but it's better to spend a bit of money for the sake of your health than to make yourself ill for the sake of a few pounds. Eye tests are free to diabetics and to those over the age of sixty.

# 5

# Shock and Stress

---

*Lynne's Mum's Story*

> *I consider myself an expert on sex, love and health.*
> *Without health, you can have very little of the other two.*
> Barbara Cartland

I've read that stress cannot cause diabetes, because if that were the case, every stressed-out person would be diabetic. However, it's well known among diabetics themselves that severe shock can kick-start diabetes in someone who is predisposed to it.

> **All diabetics know that day-to-day stress makes the disease harder to control, once they have it.**

*Lynne's Mum's Story*

Lynne sent me this piece about her mother, and I haven't cut or changed it. Lynne says that everyone concerned is dead, so nobody can be hurt by the story being aired now.

"Whilst working as a cashier in a large department store in Cardiff, Bette, aged 24, accepted an invitation for a date with a dashing young colleague. The evening went well, as they met up and enjoyed a drink in one of Cardiff's popular nightspots, and then they saw a film at the local cinema. He was charming, so she relaxed and had fun.

Her date accompanied her home, walking her to her front door and delivered what she assumed to be a goodnight kiss before making arrangements for a future rendezvous, but she noticed that he was lingering and his mood changing. His attentions became more amorous, and then aggressive.

As she found herself struggling to free herself from his tight grasp, she purposely leaned on the doorbell, knowing her parents would still be up. The doorbell rang, but her Mum assumed it was accidental - two young lovebirds fooling around in the porch.

When he realised what she had done, his behaviour worsened, and dragging her out of the porch and away from the house, he slapped and punched her and proceeded to pull her around the side of the terraced row of houses onto a deserted field. As Bette struggled frantically, her heeled dance shoe became dislodged, and as he pushed her down on the grass, her head landed on the shoe. She became quieter and waited for her chance. When it came, she reached behind her head, grasped the shoe and then used it to hit her assailant. After a few blows, he fled.

The shock of seeing Bette walk through the door, battered and bleeding, triggered type 2 diabetes in her mother, Alice, while the after effects of the attack brought on type 1 diabetes in Bette. She later described the feeling of something "snapping" in her pancreatic region, though any injury there was never confirmed.

Bette reported the incident to the manager of the store, and the man was instantly dismissed. The police were called, but Bette never pressed charges."

# 6

# Types of Diabetes

*A Serious Misconception ~ Varieties of Diabetes ~ Pre Diabetes ~ Type 2 Diabetes ~ Childhood Type 2 Diabetes and Obesity ~ Childhood Type 2 Diabetes Without Obesity ~ Type 1 Diabetes ~ Type 1.5 Diabetes ~ Type 1 and Type 2 in one Package*

> *The desire to take medicine is perhaps the greatest feature that distinguishes man from animals.*
> Sir William Osler

**There are now over 2.3 million diabetics in the UK, and about 750,000 walking around with some level of undiagnosed diabetes.**

### A Serious Misconception

Some of those who have written books on diabetes have clearly taken information from one particularly well-respected book, which for the most part is excellent, but which has accidentally put forward one really dangerous misconception. The original book and all its clones all say: "There is no such thing as mild or borderline diabetes."

When you look carefully at the original book, the writer goes on to say that diabetes is a progressive disease, and that any amount of diabetes needs to be taken seriously. Unfortunately, a combination of poor writing and lazy editing makes it sound as though one either has diabetes or one does not, and that the early stages of the ailment can happily be ignored.

Diabetics and parents of diabetics take a much more realistic view. These people severely criticise General Practitioners who tell their patients, "You have a little sugar...but it's not serious", or those who say "I see patients who have the condition in a much more severe form than you do, so stop making a fuss, and go away and forget about it." If the "lucky" patient takes this advice, his condition will soon progress to the point where he spends what's left of his life in hospital!

So now let us look at some of the forms of this strange ailment - all of which need to be taken seriously.

## *Varieties of Diabetes*

Until recently, it was considered that there were two distinct types of diabetes: type 1 and type 2. Now, we see that there are several variations on a theme, and that one can move back and forth between them, depending upon whether the disease is getting better or worse. Even type 1 diabetes can get worse, as we will soon see...

## *Pre-diabetes*

American medics call all these conditions "pre-diabetes" and thankfully, this graphically simple term is now coming into use in the UK. Other names that you might come across are:

~ Impaired glucose tolerance (IGT)
~ Impaired fasting glycaemia (IFT)
~ Diet-controlled diabetes
~ Borderline diabetes
~ Mild diabetes

Pre-diabetics usually develop type 2 diabetes within ten years of being diagnosed. Diet and exercise can keep it away for longer, so if you are pre-diabetic, the time to take action is *now!* Sadly, there are upwards of a million pre-diabetics walking around in the UK, not knowing why they feel so knackered, because they are unaware of their encroaching diabetes.

## *Type 2 Diabetes*

Type 2 diabetes occurs when the body no longer makes sufficient insulin and / or when the liver and other organs lose the ability to fully process the insulin that *is* made. This comes on gradually, usually in middle or old age. Depending upon its severity, type 2 diabetes can be treated by diet alone, with pills or with insulin. About 90 per cent of all diabetics are type 2.

## *Childhood type 2 Diabetes and Obesity*

Type 2 diabetes used to be called "mature onset diabetes" or "late onset diabetes", but now doctors in Britain and the USA are seeing children and young people with type 2, due to obesity.

## *Childhood type 2 Diabetes Without Obesity*

Diabetes can be kick-started in childhood even when a child is skinny. An ailment such as jaundice/hepatitis, added to shock and trauma, can put the child on the road to diabetes. Most children in this situation go down with type 1 diabetes, but some children become pre-diabetic and type 2 later.

## *Type 1.5 Diabetes*

There are people who get what appears to be late onset type 1 diabetes. The pancreas gives up producing insulin altogether, and they have to inject themselves three or four times a day. A lady in her late 50s called Patricia, and a man in his early 40s called Adam both have this condition. Patricia says that even the people in her diabetes clinic don't know whether to call her condition type 1 or type 2. Sue, in my local surgery, calls it type 1.5.

## Type 1 Diabetes

Type 1 diabetes usually starts in children or among young adults when something triggers an autoimmune reaction that shuts down the insulin-making beta cells in the pancreas. Type 1 diabetics need to inject insulin several times a day to stay alive. This is still a relatively uncommon ailment, because only about 10 per cent of all diabetics are type 1. There's no cure for this kind of diabetes yet, so it just has to be managed with insulin. There are alternatives to injections being investigated, but insulin can't be swallowed, because it is a hormone and a protein, and it would be digested like any other protein. Inhalant insulin experiments are being conducted, successfully, but side effects such as lung disorders still have to be fully assessed.

Type 1 diabetics must get medical help and keep on getting it, and you must read books that contain more technical information about how to use insulin and other drugs and the timing of medication and foods. You also need to join Diabetes UK.

## Type 1 and Type 2 Diabetes in One Package

Unbelievably, medicine is now turning up people who have both type 1 and type 2 diabetes at the same time! How can this be?

If a child develops type 1 diabetes, the beta glands in his pancreas stop producing insulin, so he must get daily requirements from insulin injections. The child grows up, but doesn't bother to eat carefully and he takes no exercise. He gains far too much weight, so his liver and other organs lose the ability to process the insulin that he injects. He then becomes type 2 in addition to being type 1. This is hard to treat successfully.

# 7

# My Story

---

*When Did my Problem Start? ~ Symptoms*

> *The people who say they don't have time to*
> *take care of themselves will soon discover*
> *they're spending all their time being sick.*

Patricia Alexander

### *When Did my Problem Start?*

I had a horrible childhood right from the start, both at home and at school, but things got worse after my father died. At the age of eight I began to lose the will to live, and a year later I landed up in hospital. I was filthy dirty and stick-thin from malnutrition and misery, abuse and neglect. I had seven massive sties on my eyes and raging yellow jaundice. Interestingly, I also had a wound on my foot that wouldn't heal. As the years went by, I discovered that if I scraped myself badly, the wound would take a long time to heal and scrapes often became septic.

My mother-in-law had spent forty years working in a chemist's shop, so she knew a great deal about health. I was nineteen when she first met me, and almost from the start, she suspected that I was diabetic. When I was twenty, she sent me for a blood test. The test might well have shown intolerance to glucose, but nobody told patients anything in those days, so I don't know what, if anything, showed up. However, I went on to have two children without developing gestational diabetes.

On one occasion, I remember going to London to meet my husband for a trip to the cinema. I had rushed straight from work without stopping to eat and there was a long queue at the cinema. While standing there; I started to feel very strange. It was a cool evening, but I felt sweaty, sick and peculiar. As I got older, I got used to these "funny turns" and I learned that they were due to unstable levels of blood sugar. Apart from trying to eat regularly, I didn't know what to do about it.

As I moved into early middle age, I felt increasingly unwell, and a friend suggested that I was "on the change" and that I should consult a homeopath. The homeopath said that my fatigue, misery and terrific thirst didn't gibe with the menopause, but that it sounded far more like diabetes. He asked me if there was any diabetes in my family. (There's plenty.) He gave me a blood test and explained that my blood glucose was above the normal level. He advised me on diet and said that if I took care of myself, I could stave off full diabetes for many years.

Apart from the original advice from the homeopath, no medical person suggested that I do anything special, but experience showed me that if I ate a lot of sweet stuff, I became tired and thirsty; and that my feet would burn and tingle. By my late 50s, the combination of a hysterectomy, stopping smoking, a sedentary job and getting older meant that I gained weight.

Since then, I've lost some of the weight and I eat as much fruit, salad and vegetables as I can. Most of the time, I'm fine, but it's getting harder as I get older.

### *Symptoms*

Here are some of the things that have bothered me over the years, although it's only when researching this book that I realised their implications:

~ Thrush and cystitis.
~ Thirst and dry mouth.
~ Frequent loo visits.

~ It's becoming more difficult to lose weight (typical of type 2 diabetes).

~ Dental problems turn to abscesses.

~ Colds can go on my chest if I'm not careful.

~ I get tired easily.

~ Hypoglycaemia.

~ Tingling and sometimes jabbing pains in my feet.

~ Tingling in my palms.

~ If I cut my finger, it takes an age to heal, and I once lost feeling in the end of my little finger for several months.

~ Blurred vision, sore eyes.

~ Temporary loss of sight in one eye due to stress, migraine and diabetes.

~ I can get zits, styes and my hair falls out when I don't keep my blood sugar down.

# 8

# Symptoms

---

*Symptoms ~ Worse Than Mere Symptoms ~ Hypoglycaemia*

> *A healthy body is a guest chamber for the soul;*
> *a sick body is a prison.*

Francis Bacon

### Symptoms

While I'm aware that some really nasty problems can develop when diabetes gets out of hand, I will focus on the common symptoms that affect most diabetics and pre-diabetics. Many of you will recognise them from your own experiences.

Interestingly, there are many individuals who become diabetic with no warning symptoms at all - or perhaps they get them, but don't recognise them for what they are.

> Apparently the root of the word diabetes comes from the ancient Greek, and it means siphon. The full name is diabetes mellitus. Mellitus is Latin for sweetness, so the name arises because ancient doctors discovered that a diabetic's urine tastes sweet. One wonders how they discovered this!

~ It has long been known that diabetics get thirsty, drink a lot and then pee a lot. Often, the diabetic actually seems to pee out more than he drinks in, because the body is desperate to get rid of excess glucose from the kidneys and blood, and the kidneys enlarge and then push out loads more fluid. Frequent visits to the loo during the night are common.

~ Fatigue is a symptom of many ailments, but diabetics (and near-diabetics) get seriously knackered. This is obviously worse if you can't get a good night's sleep due to frequent loo visits. Don't fill your life up with duties and don't fill your children's lives up with "activities". If you have a new baby, take a rest whenever the baby sleeps. If you're an older person and you get tired during the late afternoon, take a nap. If you suddenly feel lively at two in the morning and you feel like cooking, cleaning or working on the computer, and if it won't disturb anyone else, that's what you should do. Normality goes out of the window with this ailment, so do whatever works for you, even if it is unconventional.

~ Many people suffer from tingling and burning in the toes and soles of the feet, especially at night. When the disease gets worse, there are stabbing pains along the nerves in the feet.

~ Patches of skin on the arms and legs can feel as though someone has taken an emery board to them, but when you look, there's nothing to see. This can indicate kidney damage.

~ Vision gets blurred, because the eyes respond to changes in the levels of blood glucose. Glucose levels rise and decrease more widely and faster than in normal people, thus the eye's response sometimes lags behind. The blurring can clear up when the sugar level is better. You may notice that you can see to read, but that you struggle to see into the distance.

~ Other eye problems that are made worse by diabetes are glaucoma, cataracts and retinopathy.

~ Here's something you won't find in the medical books: A combination of diabetes and migraine, added to stress, will cause temporary blindness.

~ The mouth can be dry, the breath can smell bad and the skin can taste of honey.

~ If a person is seriously ill with insulin dependent diabetes that isn't properly controlled, ketoacidosis can occur. When this happens, the person's breath smells of rotten apples or acetone (nail lacquer remover). This can become a serious condition that is most likely to happen when a diabetic person is ill or under great stress. Detailed symptoms and measures to take are outlined on the major diabetes websites, and a quick search of the Internet will bring up many articles on this subject. One thing that is usually needed is for the person to drink copious amounts of water. This can be a good start while checking further, but usually, an urgent visit to your nearest A & E is advisable.

~ Some men find it difficult to get a full erection - although some manage well enough with only a half-hearted one and a lot of skill. Others don't have any problem with erections.

~ Both men and women can get thrush or cystitis.

~ It's hard for the body to fight infection and tooth decay. Chest infections linger.

~ Anything that happens to the feet takes an age to heal, and athlete's foot takes on a life of its own.

~ Cuts, scrapes and blisters on feet and hands don't heal easily.

~ Headaches. These can happen when the blood sugar level sinks too low, but it's also often a result of dehydration.

~ Unexplained vomiting can be a sign that pre-diabetes is turning into type 2. If you get what appears to be severe food poisoning when everyone around you had the same meal and were fine, check your blood sugar level.

~ Polycystic ovaries can be a sign of encroaching diabetes.

~ Some people break out in zits or styes.

~ Brownish crusty things can appear on the skin. Dab a bit of H45 cream on them and they will go away again. You can buy this cream over the counter. One word of warning though; seriously nasty crusts that suddenly appear on the breasts can be a symptom of cancer, so those always need to be checked out. Whitish, slightly wet crusts on the head or back can be solar keratosis, which is an early stage of skin cancer, so take these seriously too.

~ When sugar levels are high, your hair may start to fall out.

~ If there's a mosquito, gnat or midge within five miles of me, it will seek me out and bite me. Does the sweet taste of my skin attract them? I haven't asked other diabetics about this, but it would be interesting to find out.

~ Diabetics get irritable and their emotions can be up and down. Some act very weirdly if they become hypoglycaemic.

~ Many diabetics get miserable because they can't eat what they fancy. Take a tip from an old saying: "If you can't get what you want, want what you get".

~ You may not feel pain as much as others do, and something can get out of hand before you realise it.

~ Too much alcohol can cause or worsen stabbing nerve pains in the feet, ankles and shins.

~ Apparently, more diabetics suffer from Alzheimer's and Parkinson's than non-diabetics.

### Worse Than Mere Symptoms

In its worst form, diabetes is a silent and deadly killer. It thickens the blood with cholesterol, thus bringing on a heart attack or a stroke. It thickens the blood vessels in the kidneys, thus preventing the body from being able to eliminate waste. Hands and feet lose their ability to feel pain, so that an unnoticed rub or puncture on a foot causes an ulcer that can become gangrenous. In some cases, a leg has to come off at the knee just to save the patient's life. The bones in the feet can become misshapen. Diabetic retinopathy causes blindness.

**Interestingly, an American survey has found that the majority of amputees are smokers as well as being diabetic.**

## *Hypoglycaemia*

Hypoglycaemia occurs when the glucose level falls too low. The glucose level fluctuates much more in diabetics than in normal people, especially when they get older. It's a particular problem for those on pills or insulin, because these lower the glucose level artificially. Once the glucose level starts to sink, it can keep dropping for over sixteen hours without a break; this can put the diabetic into a coma, which is why some diabetics die in their sleep.

A hypo (as it's called) feels dreadful. If you take pills for your diabetes, it's essential that you learn about hypos and what to do about them. The main thing is to eat regularly, and never drink alcohol on an empty stomach, even if you control your diabetes by diet alone. Remember that extra exercise or a very busy day at work will lower the glucose level. Carry some glucose sweets on you so that you can restore your glucose level quickly if needs be, then have a biscuit or sandwich as soon as possible, and ensure that the next couple of meals contain plenty of carbohydrates, such as pasta or potatoes. In extreme cases, a tip from an experienced diabetic for swift recovery is to drink some ordinary Coca Cola. None of the other colas work as fast, and naturally, you mustn't use the diet variety! This isn't a bit of Coke promo, it's a genuine, practical piece of advice for times when swift action may be necessary.

Ensure that your family, colleagues, friends and companions and even quite young children know what the signs are and what to do about it, and wear a MedicAlert type of bracelet or necklace.

Be sure to find out more about hypos from books and from your medical team. Where diabetes is concerned, knowledge is power.

9

# Measurements and Spikes

*A Near Death Experience ~ Modern Measurements ~ Don't use Other People's Equipment ~ Useful Tips ~ Magic Numbers ~ the USA and Canada ~ How Often should you Test your Blood? ~ Spikes ~ the Tale of Three Croissants ~ Stress Levels ~ Alternatives ~ Grams and Millilitres ~ Cigareeets and Whisky and Wild, Wild Women ~*

> *I won't eat oysters. I want my food dead.*
> *Not sick, not wounded, dead.*

Woody Allen

### A Near Death Experience

There are various ways of measuring the level of glucose in the body. My grandpa used to measure his "water" several times a day with a little paper urine strip. If the paper changed colour, it registered that there was too much glucose in the urine. The density of the colour showed roughly how much glucose there was. I gather that these "pee-sticks" only start to react when there's something like 14 mmol/l of blood glucose, and that is already far too much, as that's twice the level one would like to see.

I bought these sticks in the past, but I never saw any reaction on them - apart from once. I peed on the stick and then looked at it. To my horror, it was dead black, signifying that my glucose level was so high that I was in imminent danger of dying! I picked another stick out of the little pot with the intention of trying again as soon as I could rustle up some more pee. As soon as the stick came out of the pot, I noticed that it was also black - and nobody had piddled on that one yet! I picked up the pot and looked inside. All the sticks were black. Apparently, the lid had come slightly undone, the sticks had got damp and that had made them react. So, look after your testing equipment carefully, no matter what kind you use.

### Modern Measurements

A home blood testing kit needs only a teeny-tiny spot of blood on a special paper stick to make the measurement. Home blood testing kits are very sensitive, so they measure blood glucose accurately enough for most purposes.

If you become medically defined as a diabetic and need to take medication, you will be able to get the strips on prescription. That is a great help, as they are currently about £26 for 50 strips.

Don't change your tester if you are happy with it. There may be a new all-singing-and-dancing model on the market, but there's no need to buy it if you are happy with your present model.

### Don't Use Other People's Equipment

Caroline was recently diagnosed with type 2 diabetes and she mentioned this to Lauren. Lauren's mother-in-law has diabetes, and the old lady had a couple of old testing machines lying around, so Lauren rushed hot-foot over to Caroline with one of her mother-in-law's old testers. After a good deal of bossy advice about what to eat, and general "I know best-ing", Lauren tested Caroline's blood and announced to Caroline that her blood glucose measured 2.2 mmol/l! Caroline told us about this the next day and we laughed - a person with this low a level would be seriously and visibly hypo! It was obvious that either the tester was completely clapped out or that the test strips were not properly calibrated to match the tester.

Caroline now has her own tester and she keeps an eye on her own situation.

## Disposal

Take care to dispose of your testing materials carefully. The best thing is probably to burn the used blood strips in an open fire or to burn them in a pot in the garden, but if you can't do that, put them in a bag and then into the bin. Always put the little cap back on the lancet after you have used it, before throwing it out.

## Neurosis

If you have only recently become diabetic, you might be a bit neurotic at the start, testing yourself every hour or so. New diabetics who are on pills may test themselves very frequently, and then get the wind up when the levels fluctuate at various times of the day. Some can drive their GPs nuts, running round to the surgery on a daily basis and asking if they should take more pills on some days and fewer on others. Fortunately, it's human nature to get used to things and it's even more human to tire of things, so, even if you start out being thoroughly neurotic about your blood glucose tests, you will soon settle down into a suitable routine.

Depending upon the type and severity of the diabetes, people test themselves anything from several times a day to just a couple of times a month. I test my blood every week, unless I feel weird, and then I will do an extra check.

*Here are some useful tips:*

~ Do the test before putting hand cream on your hands, or you won't get a proper reading. Wash your hands in warm water before pricking your finger.

~ When taking a blood test, prick the sides of the fingers rather than the tips as this hurts less. Having said that, modern lancets are pretty painless.

~ Use the lowest setting that will draw the smallest amount of blood that you need and you will hardly feel it.

~ If the blood doesn't want to flow, hang your hands down and rub them together as if you were washing them.

~ Don't pinch the finger to get blood out, as you will end up with a mixture of blood, body fluid and perspiration, which may give a false reading.

~ If blood really doesn't want to flow, put a rubber band around the base of the finger - and remember to take it off again when you've finished.

~ Never use the same lancet twice, and never share a needle with someone else.

~ When you've finished, put the cap back on the lancet before throwing it into the dustbin.

You don't always have to use your fingers for the test - they are convenient, but if you wish to use your thigh or other reasonable places on your body. The drawback is that these places don't register changes in glucose levels as quickly as the fingers do. You'll probably find guidance on good areas included in the machine's instruction leaflet.

Most specialists recommend testing every hour or so in specific circumstances, such as when performing extreme sports or strenuous, continuous activities. These situations are so delicate and complex that they demand specific knowledge - so if you want to train for the Olympics or any strenuous sports, please take specialist advice first, and all along the way. Normal type 2 diabetics may only need to test themselves once every week or two, unless there's a temporary reason for them to test more often, say after eating something unusual.

If more precise tests are needed, these are done at the surgery, clinic or at a special unit in a hospital. The most common is a "fasting" test, where you will be asked to avoid eating and drinking (apart from water) for twelve hours beforehand. The test is usually done first thing in the morning. This is called an HbA1c test, which measures the glucose in the blood plasma. The test is done once, and then again about three months later. This will show how much sugar has stuck to the red blood cells and it will also show the general level of glucose in the blood during that time.

A glucose tolerance test is done at a diabetic clinic. You have a blood test and then drink a special liquid, sit around for two hours and then have a second blood test. This shows how well your body has tolerated the glucose drink.

You can read about these tests in detail in the books I've listed in the bibliography at the back of this book.

*Magic Numbers for Home Testing*

The following data comes from Diabetes UK and it covers the different types of test for blood glucose, blood pressure, cholesterol and size.

*Levels for Blood, Fats, and Waistline*

**Ideal blood glucose levels. Aim for these at all times:**
4-6 mmol/l before meals, and up to 10 mmol/l two hours after
   meals. The reading may be higher first thing in the morning.

**Acceptable blood glucose levels that show problems, but not yet a medical emergency:**
4-7 mmol/l before meals, and up to 11 mmol/l two hours after
   meals.

**HbA1c:**
Below 6.5% in most cases, but below 7% in all cases.

**Blood pressure:**
Below 130/80.

**Blood fats:**
Triglyceride level 1.7 mmol/l or less.
Total cholesterol less than 4.5 mmol/l.

**Waist measurement:**
White and black men: less than 37 inches.
Asian men: less than 35 inches.
White and black women: less than 31.5 inches.
Asian women: Less than 31.5 inches.

Modern home blood testing machines keep a record of your tests, but it makes sense to keep a "diary" for your own benefit, and also to show a doctor or nurse when the need arises. Make up something like this on a computer or by hand, and make enough photocopies for your needs:

| DATE | TIME | MMOL/L | STOMACH |
|------|------|--------|---------|
| 1st Jan | 3 pm | 6.9 | Half empty |
| 7th Jan | 10 am | 6.5 | Half empty |
| 15th Jan | 8 pm | 8.2 | Full |
| 22nd Jan | 12 noon | 5.5 | Empty *(feeling hypo-ish)* |
| 30th Jan | 8 am | 7.7 | Empty |
| 6th Feb | 2 pm | 8.4 | Full |

**Your reading may be higher first thing in the morning, even though you haven't yet eaten or drunk anything. The explanation is that the body thinks that it's fasting (not having eating for a few hours), so it releases more glucose.**

**Exercise may lift your reading temporarily, because the body will have released extra glucose to help the muscles produce energy while you're doing your thing. However, the overall long-term effect of exercise is good.**

## The USA and Canada

Years ago, I had a diabetic American friend, and he commented that my blood glucose measurement was weird, while I thought his was meaningless. Mine was something like eight at the time, while his was something like 150! The reason for the discrepancy is that where home blood testing machines are concerned, the US uses a system of mg/dl, which refers to milligrams per decilitre. To convert ours to theirs, multiply by 18 and to convert theirs to ours, divide by 18.

*How Often Should You Test Your Blood?*

There's a huge variation in frequency from person to person and from one type of diabetic to another. The need also depends upon what you happen to be doing at any specific moment in time. Here are some variations upon a theme:

Some doctors aren't in favour of home testing, because they think it encourages patients to become neurotic and demanding.

Many medical staff try to keep costs down by discouraging testing and thus saving on the paper strips that are used. If your practice suffers from terminal stinginess, buy a pot of strips for yourself. They cost about 50p per strip, but it is your life that's on the line, so the expenditure is worth it.Strips may be a little cheaper when you buy them over the Internet, but be sure to use a reliable, accredited source. All the books I've read recommend frequent testing, especially for type 1 diabetics and for type 2's whose diabetes is hard to control.

~ If you're a type 2 diabetic, you're eating the right things, taking some exercise and you feel fine, then a test every seven to ten days is probably fine.
~ If you feel lousy: test!
~ If you eat something unusual and want to be sure of the results: test after eating, and again two hours later.
~ If you're about to embark on some unusually heavy or sustained activity, test before you start, stop and test while doing it and test again immediately afterwards and then again a couple of hours later. If you're on medication or insulin, this is essential, in addition to taking advice and instructions from your medical advisor.

Regardless of what your friends or anybody else might say, you should do what feels right to you. You may not wish to divulge the results of your tests to your doctor or anyone else, and you're not obliged to. You are the one with the diabetes, and you know how you feel and what you need to do. Even if your doctor and all your friends are also diabetic, they may not have the same kind of diabetes as you do, or theirs may not be at the same stage as yours. You must take charge of your own life, and that starts by knowing what is or isn't going on inside your blood stream. Conversely, if you have a pal who tests seventeen times a day, but you feel perfectly comfortable testing once a fortnight, that's fine. If I feel fine, I test about once a week, but if I feel the need, I test every day for a while.

Just remember that:
(a) You may need first aid, for example, after an accident where you lose consciousness, or if you slip into a hypo coma. Anyone treating you really ought to know about your diabetes before they apply the wrong treatment.
(b) You do have a responsibility to others; if there's a possibility of you causing harm to others - if, for example, your vision deteriorates to the extent that you shouldn't be driving, then you have to act appropriately.

If you inject insulin and you drive a car, you are obliged by law to advise the DVLA of your condition. If your are on medication, you are also meant to advise the DVLA. Check the details from time to time, as legislation may change. Furthermore, if you don't declare a medical condition properly, then you'll find that filing a successful insurance claim becomes rather difficult...

## *Spikes*
If you eat something that makes you "spike" higher than expected, take a brisk walk around the block, keep sipping water for a couple of hours and visit the loo every time your bladder fills. It's hard to cope with all this while you're out shopping or at work, so I suggest that you avoid eating the things that push your glucose level up when you're out and about. If you want to experiment with foods, do it at home, where you can undo the damage fairly quickly. Keep a couple

of small bottles of water in the car for when you travel, along with biscuits and coca cola for hypos.

## Spikes, or the Tale of Three Croissants

I love croissants, so one day when I was hungry, I ate three of them in a row. I decided to see how that affected me, so I left it for an hour and then did a blood test. Sure enough, it registered over 11 mmol/l. That is a hell of a lot of millimoles for someone who - technically - is a diet-controlled type 2 diabetic!

I drank water, used the loo, went for a walk, drank more water and used the loo again, and soon the level was down to 6.4 mmol/l. If you're a type 2 diabetic rather than a pre-diabetic like me, you will spike higher than this, and find it harder to bring the level down again, so be careful. I now only buy one croissant at a time.

## Stress Levels

Some doctors say that stress doesn't cause diabetes, but if you're already diabetic or pre-disposed to it, stress will make it hard for you to keep your glucose level down. Those who work in alternative and complementary therapies always consider that a person's mental and spiritual condition contributes to an ailment. Some take this too far and attribute every ailment to stress. Diabetes is caused by a mechanical fault in the body, but stress definitely makes it harder for the body to cope with it.

## Alternatives

If you're into spiritual or alternative healing and if you understand the chakra system, you should ask for healing for your Solar Plexus Chakra. Alternative healing is often very calming and relaxing, so it's worth pursuing this as an aid and a backup to any conventional treatment you're receiving. Never let anyone talk you into relying solely on complementary therapies, or on using them in place of conventional treatment. Avoid the kind of complementary treatment that puts something into your body, and this includes homeopathy, aromatherapy and herbal medicine, all of which introduce materials into the body. Always tell your complementary therapist about your conventional medical treatment. A magnetic bracelet can help to improve blood flow through the body, and it can ease aches and pains

You don't usually need to tell your doctor about things that are non-invasive, such as massage, reflexology, crystal healing, spiritual healing and so on. All these help the body's ability to heal, to relax, to make full use of its immune system and to fight diabetes.

## *Grams and Millilitres*

When we talk about the contents of cans, packets, jars and bottles, most measurements in the UK are in grams, and it's the grams of sugar per hundred grams that you need to measure. Liquid measurements are in litres or perhaps millilitres, and it's the millilitres per hundred millilitres that you want to check on.

## *Cigareeets and Whisky and Wild, Wild Women*

There used to be a popular cowboy song that went, "Cigareeets and whisky and wild, wild women will drive you crazy and drive you insane-ane-ane!" Well, can they?

Years ago I used to smoke and I loved every fag I ever inhaled, and I never came across a bad one - not even those smelly French things - but I decided to give it up before it gave me up. Smoking has a peculiar effect on the strangest parts of the body, including the veins, arteries, kidneys and bladder. In diabetes, the kidneys and bladder are not in the best of health to start with, so they don't need the toxins in tobacco smoke on top of everything else.

The good news is that you can drink a little alcohol with diabetes (wey, hey!), but not every kind of alcohol is recommended. If you're seriously ill or if you're advised not to drink, then don't!

### My Research Findings on Alcohol

Most type 2 diabetics can drink a little. Some sources say that a diabetic can drink up to the recommended minimum of 14 units a week for women and 21 units a week for men, but in reality this is too much. It's better to drink a little on two or three evenings a week than to go out once in a month and get paralytic.

If you take pills or use insulin injections, adding alcohol to the mix can be a very dangerous combination, due to too great a drop in blood sugar. Worse still, a hypo makes a person appear drunk, so a diabetic who is out on the town with his friends can become seriously ill and even die, because his companions don't realise that he may be dangerously hypoglycaemic. Blood sugar can keep on dropping for up to 16 hours after drinking, so in extreme circumstances, a diabetic could die while asleep after a night out on the tiles.

Alcohol makes the pain in the feet that is caused by nerve damage much worse, and it can affect the eyes badly as well. Heavy drinking damages the liver, and the liver is needed to process insulin. Alcohol can raise the level of triglycerides that cause artery and heart disease, so if you have a cholesterol problem or any other problem that doesn't mix well with drink, consider not drinking at all.

Frankly, if you feel that you can't get through life without drinking - even if you aren't a heavy drinker - it might be worth attending Alcoholics Anonymous.

### Wild, Wild Women - and Wild, Wild Men

These are definitely recommended for all diabetics, because "exercise" lowers your blood glucose levels!

---

**Improve your knowledge by reading other books about diabetes. Ask your medical specialist for advice.**

# 10

# Diabetes and Sugars

*The Distant Past ~ The Recent Past ~ the Present ~ Commercially Prepared Foods ~ The Question and the Answer ~ Diabetic Products ~ Sweeteners ~ A Warning ~ Fruit Sugar ~ Problems?*

> *Jack and Jill went into town*
> *To fetch some chips and sweeties*
> *He can't keep his heart rate down*
> *And she's got diabetes!*

Anonymous writer

### The Distant Past

Years ago, not only did diabetics have to do without sugar entirely, but their intake of all carbohydrates was severely restricted. They worked on a series of "exchanges", where they exchanged a slice of wholemeal bread at a meal for one small potato or three ounces of uncooked pasta. This made diabetics so hungry that they cheated or filled up on meats and fatty foods. Some, like my grandpa, smoked panatela cigars all day to keep the hunger pangs at bay. As it happens, Grandpa didn't lose any limbs or his eyesight, and he lived to his mid-seventies, which wasn't bad for his generation, but the last few years of his life were uncomfortable because he developed a weak heart due to his diabetes.

### The Recent Past

Michael was a type 1 diabetic who coped by injecting insulin and then eating Chinese takeaways several times a week. I once saw him watching television while working his way through a large tin of biscuits! When I asked him about this, he said that injecting with insulin meant that he didn't have to worry about what he ate. In a way, my late biscuit-eating friend had a point, because the diabetic on pills or insulin can get away with more than the diet-controlled diabetic. Unfortunately, Michael died while still in his forties. His death certificate should have read, "Died from sweet and sour pork, fried rice, prawn crackers and biscuits".

### The Present

Modern diets suggest limiting sugar but not eliminating it entirely, so these now allow for an occasional cake and even an occasional piece of chocolate. Diabetic cookbooks even show some recipes that use sugar or honey.

GPs prefer to advise patients to avoid sweet foods altogether, so they will suggest that the patient never eats cake, dessert, ice cream, sweets, chocolates and so on. Why? They know human nature, and they know that what comes out of their mouths as, "An occasional plain biscuit or bit of cake is all right" goes into the patient's ears as, "Stuff your face with a family-sized chocolate gâteau three times a week".

Similarly, the modern view is that salad dressings, ketchup, pickles and sauces are fine, because we don't eat much of these in one sitting, but almost every meal contains something of this kind, so why not select those that are lower in sugar? If you look at the labels on things and choose those that contain up to 6g of sugar in 100g, you will still eat nice things, but without accumulating unnecessary sugar in your system.

### Commercially Prepared Foods

You can't avoid eating sugar altogether, because so many everyday products contain it, so I suggest that you keep a close eye on what's inside everything that you buy. Look at the label on the back of the packet, can, pot, bottle or whatever that you buy, and check where it shows the contents per 100 grams. That's exactly what the labelling is for, so use the information! Until your glucose level is steady and/or you have lost weight, try to keep everything that you buy for yourself below 6 grams per 100 grams. For the most part, swapping one make of something for another isn't that difficult. For example, some mayonnaise and salad dressings can contain over 17g of sugar per 100g, while other makes have less than 6g per 100g. Caesar salad dressing and blue cheese dressing taste nice and they both contain less than 6g of sugars per 100g.

Your first couple of visits to the supermarket will take you a half a day, but after that, you will soon learn. Once you know what to buy, type up a shopping list for yourself, make lots of copies, and leave copies in your pocket, in your shopping bag in your car, or in your bike's basket. Then you'll have your list to hand at all times. The writing on the back of tins, jars and packets is often small and written in colours that make it hard to read, so, if it helps, take a magnifying glass along when you go shopping.

It's no good telling yourself that you never eat processed foods, because unless you have your own personal shopper and cook who has nothing else to do all day but prepare excellent foods for you, you do. Even cheese is processed, as are most ham and other "deli" foods, and the same goes for many other things.

---

**There's no particular need for diabetics to choose organic foods, but you may wish to do so for all-round good health.**

---

**Be careful: commercially made "healthy option" foods are often just smaller portions of normal foods.**

### The Question and the Answer

**Question:** What is the difference between a diabetic cake recipe and a normal cake recipe?

**Answer:** The special recipes for diabetics contain more fibre and less sugar, salt and fat than normal ones do.

**Question:** Is a homemade cake better than a shop-bought one?
**Answer:** Yes, because you know exactly what's in it.

### Diabetic Products

Most diabetic books tell you never to buy special diabetic foods such as jam, biscuits, sweets and chocolate, because they are expensive, fattening, not good for diabetes, and full of things that give you diarrhoea. I remember a recently diagnosed type 2 friend who ate his way through a diabetic Easter egg and spent the rest of the holidays tied to the loo! Diabetic jam tastes bitter and gives you dreadful wind and diarrhoea. Better to eat a little reduced-sugar jam or even ordinary jam, but spread it on very sparingly. However, there are times when a dia-biscuit can save your sanity.

### Sweeteners

Splenda is made from sucralose (a product of sugar), but it's fine.

Canderel etc. contain aspartame / acesulfame, and these are ok to add to hot drinks, fruit or _cooked_ food.

### Warning

Although advertised as being suitable for cooking or baking, there are also sources advising that high temperatures cause aspartame to release chemicals, such as formalin, that damage the nerves. It also loses much of its sweetness when heated in this way. I have to mention that there is much debate about artificial sweeteners generally. It is difficult to establish whether or not they / any of them are in fact completely safe, and I can only assume that in reasonable amounts, they should be reasonably safe. It's advisable to keep up to date via the Internet and organisations such as Diabetes UK.

## *Fruit Sugar*

Some packs of fruit sugar say that the contents are suitable for diabetics. This kind of sugar turns to glucose five times more slowly than other types of sugar, and it's sweeter than sugar so you only need a little of it. This will, nevertheless, add glucose to your blood, so use it sparingly.

## *Problems?*

If you're constipated, eat apples, prunes and some All Bran breakfast cereal. If you have diarrhoea, eat more eggs than you normally do and make mashed potato with skimmed milk or other soft foods that don't irritate the bowel. If you get a real stomach upset, this is a good old remedy that really works. Every two hours or so, drink a half a glass of still spring water with half a lemon squeezed into it, with a couple of Canderel dropped in, to make it palatable. In this case, Canderel is preferable to Splenda!

---

**In many countries, even in the USA, food isn't labelled the way it is here, so if you are on a self-catering holiday overseas, take great care. Americans have a very sweet tooth, so there is sugar in the most surprising foods.**

# 11

# Diabetes and Fats

---

*Fat and Cholesterol ~ Meat and Fat ~ Dairy Foods ~ Fish
~ Eggs ~ Fried Food ~ Home Grown Cholesterol*

> *The first law of dietetics seems to be:
> "if it tastes good, it's bad for you".*

Isaac Asimov

As recently as a dozen years ago, the advice given in
diabetes clinics was to eliminate sugar and severely restrict
carbohydrates. The outcome of route was that diabetics took
in far too much fat. A high fat diet is no good for the health
of a normal person, but it can be lethal for a diabetic.
Modern medical advice is to eat what anyone would describe
as "a healthy diet", including fruit, salad and vegetables,
high fibre carbohydrates and reduced levels of sugar and
fats, along with a variety of foodstuffs - and even some "bad
food choices" on occasion.

## Fat and Cholesterol

You need more medical knowledge than I have, in order to
understand the different kinds of cholesterol, triglycerides and
their effects on the body. Cholesterol comes from the foods that
we eat, but our own bodies also manufacture it. There's plenty of
information about cholesterol on the Internet, and I recommend

that you look into the books that I have listed at the back of this book as well.

What I *do* know is that diabetes makes the blood "sticky", and it thickens the walls of the arteries, veins and the internal walls of some organs. This leads to high blood pressure, and to the wrong kind of cholesterol sitting around in the blood and piling up in the arteries and organs, eventually creating a heart attack or stroke. There are drugs that control cholesterol, but they don't suit everyone. If you can lower your cholesterol by controlling your diet and taking some exercise, this can only help your general health and your diabetes.

The biggest sources of bad cholesterols are in fats such as goose fat, chicken fat, beef dripping and lard, sausages, meat, processed, fried and dairy foods.

Trans fats, which are also called homogenised or partially homogenised fats are vegetable oils that have been treated with chemicals to make them solid and spread-able. This is definitely not a good thing for your body, so avoid spreads, peanut butter and other things that contain hydrogenated fat or oil.

Good cholesterol goes through the arteries and veins like a bottlebrush, cleaning all the sticky muck off them as they go. This is found in olive oil, sunflower oil, rapeseed oil, nuts, seeds and dried apricots. There are lots of seeds in granary bread and "seedy" bread. Avocados are a source of good oils.

> **Always tell your dentist about any drugs that you're taking, as some blood pressure and cholesterol drugs don't mix well with dental drugs.**

### Meat and Fat

Buy the leanest meat that you can find, avoiding fatty cuts of bacon and those ready-prepared rolls of lamb-belly with stuffing. If someone serves you a portion of meat that has visible fat on it, cut the fat off. Even when you can't see fat, it's threaded in and out of the meat and that makes the meat tasty, so only eat meaty meals (beef, pork, lamb and ham) two or three times a week.

Pies, pasties and so on are a real problem, because you don't know exactly what is in them, but fat and some kind of starchy filler are likely to be there, and if you consider the pastry alone without any contents, it holds a lot of fat.

Deli foods are nearly all meaty and fatty. For instance, salami is lovely, but you can actually see the lumps of fat looking back at you from the plate, so don't eat this too often. This includes the pepperoni in pizza, because that is also salami. Pâté, liver sausage and meat pastes are mainly fat with a little meat added. These products remind me of the ancient Weight Watcher's saying, "if it's spread-able, its inedible!"

**There was a recent newspaper article that mentioned the possibility of a donkey sadly ending up being shipped overseas to end up in a salami factory somewhere in Europe. When my husband read this, he wanted to march round to our local supermarket immediately and demand a CSI analysis of all their salamis. My reaction was that I know horsemeat is low in cholesterol, so if donkey meat is similar, it could be a healthy option. You should have seen my husband's face! To the best of my knowledge, the UK doesn't import horsy products for human consumption...**

Deer, buck, antelope - or whatever you call things that look like Bambi - are low in cholesterol, but these animals are probably not a normal part of your shopping trolley.

Poultry is a very good option, with turkey being an excellent source of low fat food. (Pity about the bird flu, though!) Game is also good, so if you're among the wealthy few who keep quails, go grouse shooting or have a partridge in your pear tree, you have a source of healthy meat. Ostrich is probably another low-fat option, but would this be your choice for the Sunday joint?

Beef burgers are very fatty, but if you make them at home, use one of the tabletop grillers that remove a whole lot of fat.

### Dairy Foods

The jury seems to come in and go out where dairy foods are concerned. The latest thinking is that milk is actually good for the heart, but that you should choose semi-skimmed milk for most purposes, and skimmed milk for cooking. Some nutritionists are so unhappy with the contents of spreads that they advocate a return to butter. I keep my options open by varying the make of spreads that I buy, rather than buying the same one each time and I occasionally buy spread-able butter. Edam, Gouda and Brie cheeses are said to be less fattening, and there are now light and low fat versions of many other cheeses.

Cheese is quite salty and it contains milk fat. When I was a child, the only cheese that seemed to be available was very sharp Cheddar, which I hated - yet we were continually exhorted to eat cheese, as it was supposedly very good for us. Now, some American doctors call cheese junk food! As I said, the jury on cheese goes in and out. It's best to eat a variety of foods, including cheese if you like it and if it doesn't give you migraine.

### Fish

Technically speaking some fishes are fatty, but the oils in the fish are the healthy kind. There's a little cholesterol in prawns, shrimps and lobster, but nobody eats a large quantity of these foods, so they aren't worth worrying about. All told, any kind of fish is a good option, and fish, such as sardines and mackerel, contain omega 3, which is good for the heart.

### Eggs

Eggs have a bad reputation, because they contain cholesterol, but the latest thinking is that this isn't the bad kind of cholesterol that clogs your arteries. The most recent advice that I can find is that you should only eat one egg per day. Remember that many foods contain eggs, and you might have eggs as part of a meal while you're out in a café, so perhaps you should restrict yourself to no more than four or five eggs a week as home cooked meals.

I often make scrambled egg in the microwave as a better option than frying. I put two eggs per person, and a little semi-skimmed milk, along with a dash of salt and pepper into a deep bowl, and mix them thoroughly. I put the bowl into the microwave for a minute and a half, then take it out and use a fork to break up the wet, eggy mixture. I put it back into the microwave, "nuke" it for a further minute, then serve on toast.

I've tried poaching eggs in special poachers in the microwave, but this really is taking one's life in one's hands, as the closed egg holders tend explode in the microwave. I've tried larger microwave-able pots using cling film over the top, with variable results. If you like an exciting life, try this for yourself, but if your microwave is at head height, back away while it's in action, in case the door flies open and the eggs escape!

## *Fried Food*

Most people love fried food, and we all eat it from time to time. As long as you don't have too many fried meals and as long as you're not heavily overweight this is fine, but you need to choose the right kind of frying oil. My research suggests that the best choices for frying are sunflower, rapeseed and olive oils. Sunflower oil is useful for occasions when you don't want the taste of the oil to intrude, such as when frying chips, fish, stir-fry Chinese style dishes and mushrooms. If you make ratatouille or fried capsicum peppers and onions, you might choose sunflower or olive oil, depending upon your personal tastes.

Buy the extra virgin type of olive oil, as this is from the first pressing of the olives, so it's fresher and it doesn't contain any (deliberate or accidental) additives. I've tried oil from various Mediterranean countries and I find them all very nice.

Where possible, bake, microwave or grill foods, and use an electric tabletop griller for fatty foods. If you use the grill pan in your cooker, line the pan with foil and the grill with foil, then poke holes between the wires. The fat will run away from the food while keeping the wires and grill fairly clean, so that you don't have to scrape off baked-on foods afterwards.

### *Home Grown Cholesterol*

The "A-type" person is a whiz kid, a go-getter and a living success story. He finds it hard to relax and his mind is always whirring. He is competitive. Even on his holiday yacht, he can't relax, so he issues orders all day long from his BlackBerry and laptop. He has probably been divorced a few times.

> I say "he" here, because it fits the image, but there are many successful women in the world.

These people have very high standards for themselves and for others. They can be quick-tempered, abrupt, offensive and demanding. They have well-developed egos. To see several examples of this group in action, watch Dragon's Den or The Apprentice on the television. These people are obvious candidates for heart attacks or strokes.

There's another version of the choleric personality who is in even more danger of a heart attack, and this is the "wannabe A-type personality". This person wants it, but doesn't quite achieve it, so he spends much time boiling with resentment. He may have a calm or friendly outer manner, but the moiling-and-boiling goes on inside. He may make his family suffer, although outsiders never see this. Worse still, his resentment, hatreds and disappointment with others and to himself, all go on an inward journey, ending up with fatty deposits that set like concrete in his arteries. With the addition of diabetes, such a person is under sentence of an early death.

# 12

# The Techie Stuff

---

*GI: the Glycaemic Index ~ Body Mass Index ~ a Lesson in
Arithmetic ~ BMI in action ~ Shape ~ Age*

> *I eat like a vulture;*
> *Unfortunately the resemblance doesn't end there.*

Groucho Marx

## GI: The Glycaemic Index

It's amazing how language changes. Not long ago, a GI was an
American serviceman. When these young men were in Britain
during the Second World War, it was said that they were
"overpaid, oversexed and over here", but we loved them, and we
were grateful for their help. The initials "GI", I'm told, came
from the words, "Government Issue", which was stamped on
American military equipment. Now "GI" stands for "Glycaemic
Index", which is much less glamourous or romantic, but it's also
unlikely to land you up with an unwanted pregnancy!

Some foods have a high GI and others have a low GI. High
GI foods convert to glucose quickly and efficiently and should
be avoided. Low GI foods take time to digest, so they stave off
hunger and turn to glucose slowly. Interestingly, the multi-
billion pound slimming industry has jumped on the GI
bandwagon, as they have discovered that low GI foods can help
dieters to lose weight.

## *A Lesson in Arithmetic*

The Glycaemic Index is based upon the rate at which glucose is absorbed into the body, and it uses fast acting foods like white bread as the basis for the measurement. This measurement counts as 100 and everything else is measured against this number. Thus, something that is absorbed at half the rate of white bread has a GI of 50.

A diabetic should swap higher GI foods for lower ones wherever possible. Sometimes the addition of another type of food to the high GI item lowers the GI. This sounds weird and a bit potty, but here's how it works. A slice of bread or a baked potato both have a high GI, but add a bit of meat, some prawns, egg, tuna, cheese or some other form of non-carb food and the GI of the meal as a whole drops, because the average GI comes down.

It's not difficult to substitute low GI foods for high ones. Here are a few suggestions:

| HIGH GI | LOW GI |
|---|---|
| White bread | Wholegrain bread |
| Breakfast cereal | Porridge |
| Biscuits and savoury biscuits | Fruit bar thingies *(watch for added sugar though)* |
| Potatoes | Pasta, especially brown pasta |
| Old potatoes | New potatoes |
| Jacket potato | Jacket potato with tuna |
| Long grain, risotto or pudding rice | Basmati rice |
| Bananas, tropical fruit | Apples, pears, plums |
| Milk chocolate bar | Dark cooking chocolate |
| Carbohydrates (bread, pastry, rice, pasta, couscous) | Vegetables, salads, pulses, meat, fish, eggs, cheese (any protein or any food plant) |
| Any sugar, regardless of colour or type | Fruit sugar and artificial sweeteners |

## Body Mass Index (BMI)

This trendy new measurement is usually referred to as BMI. It relates to the amount of fat in your body. Not an absolutely accurate measurement, but good enough for most purposes, the BMI is calculated as follows:

### Metric Calculation for Anoraks

Your weight in kilograms (Kg) divided by your height in metres (m) squared. The formula is shown as Kg/m2, and this example shows exactly how to work it out:

Take a person's weight of 70Kg, and a height of 1.8m:
Divide 70 by (1.8 x 1.8)
BMI = 70 divided by 3.24 = 21.6

### Imperial Calculation for Anoraks

Divide your weight in pounds (lb) by the square of your height in inches (in), and then multiply by 703.
An example:
Weight: 160lb, height: 71in.
= 160 / (71 x 71) x 703
= 160 / 5,041 = 0.031739
BMI = 0.031739 x 703 = 22.3

Both of these examples show normal BMI levels.
Here are easy-to-use assessment and calculation tables, derived from www.diabetesuk.co.uk, the helpful Diabetes UK website:

| Obesity & Risk of Disease, shown by BMI and Waist Size | | | |
|---|---|---|---|
| BMI | Weight Range | Waist less than: Men - 40" (101.5cm) Women - 35" (89cm) | Waist greater than: Men - 40" (101.5cm) Women - 35" (89cm) |
| 18.4 or less | Underweight | __ | __ |
| 18.5 - 24.9 | Normal | __ | __ |
| 25.0 - 29.9 | Overweight | Increased | High |
| 30.0 - 34.9 | Obese | High | Very high |
| 35.0 - 39.9 | Very obese | Very high | Very high |
| 40 or more | Highly obese | Extremely high | Extremely high |

## *This Table is Easy to Understand and Use*

| BMI | Height (inches): 58 | 59 | 60 | 61 | 62 | 63 | 64 | 65 | 66 | 67 | 68 | 69 | 70 | 71 | 72 | 73 | 74 | 75 | 76 |
|---|---|---|---|---|---|---|---|---|---|---|---|---|---|---|---|---|---|---|---|
| | | | | | | | | | Body Weight (pounds) | | | | | | | | | | |
| 35 | 167 | 173 | 179 | 185 | 191 | 197 | 204 | 210 | 216 | 223 | 230 | 236 | 243 | 250 | 258 | 265 | 272 | 279 | 287 |
| 34 | 162 | 168 | 174 | 180 | 186 | 191 | 197 | 204 | 210 | 217 | 223 | 230 | 236 | 243 | 250 | 257 | 264 | 272 | 279 |
| 33 | 158 | 163 | 168 | 174 | 180 | 186 | 192 | 198 | 204 | 211 | 216 | 223 | 229 | 236 | 242 | 250 | 256 | 264 | 271 |
| 32 | 153 | 158 | 163 | 169 | 175 | 180 | 186 | 192 | 198 | 204 | 210 | 216 | 222 | 229 | 235 | 242 | 249 | 256 | 263 |
| 31 | 148 | 153 | 158 | 164 | 169 | 175 | 180 | 186 | 192 | 198 | 203 | 209 | 216 | 222 | 228 | 235 | 241 | 248 | 254 |
| 30 | 143 | 148 | 153 | 158 | 164 | 169 | 174 | 180 | 186 | 191 | 197 | 203 | 209 | 215 | 221 | 227 | 233 | 240 | 246 |
| 29 | 138 | 143 | 148 | 153 | 158 | 163 | 169 | 174 | 179 | 185 | 190 | 196 | 202 | 208 | 213 | 219 | 225 | 232 | 238 |
| 28 | 134 | 138 | 143 | 148 | 153 | 158 | 163 | 168 | 173 | 178 | 184 | 189 | 195 | 200 | 206 | 212 | 218 | 224 | 230 |
| 27 | 129 | 133 | 138 | 143 | 147 | 152 | 157 | 162 | 167 | 172 | 177 | 182 | 188 | 193 | 199 | 204 | 210 | 216 | 221 |
| 26 | 124 | 128 | 133 | 137 | 142 | 146 | 151 | 156 | 161 | 166 | 171 | 176 | 181 | 186 | 191 | 197 | 202 | 208 | 213 |
| 25 | 119 | 124 | 128 | 132 | 136 | 141 | 145 | 150 | 155 | 159 | 164 | 169 | 174 | 179 | 184 | 189 | 194 | 200 | 205 |
| 24 | 115 | 119 | 123 | 127 | 131 | 135 | 140 | 144 | 148 | 153 | 158 | 162 | 167 | 172 | 177 | 182 | 186 | 192 | 197 |
| 23 | 110 | 114 | 118 | 122 | 126 | 130 | 134 | 138 | 142 | 146 | 151 | 155 | 160 | 165 | 169 | 174 | 179 | 184 | 189 |
| 22 | 105 | 109 | 112 | 116 | 120 | 124 | 128 | 132 | 136 | 140 | 144 | 149 | 153 | 157 | 162 | 166 | 171 | 176 | 180 |
| 21 | 100 | 104 | 107 | 111 | 115 | 118 | 122 | 126 | 130 | 134 | 138 | 142 | 146 | 150 | 154 | 159 | 163 | 168 | 172 |
| 20 | 96 | 99 | 102 | 106 | 109 | 113 | 116 | 120 | 124 | 127 | 131 | 135 | 139 | 143 | 147 | 151 | 155 | 160 | 164 |
| 19 | 91 | 94 | 97 | 100 | 104 | 107 | 110 | 114 | 118 | 121 | 125 | 128 | 132 | 136 | 140 | 144 | 148 | 152 | 156 |

Clearly, if your details fall into the shaded area of the table, then you really need to re-assess your lifestyle and eating habits if you want to minimise and/or reduce health problems, now and in the future.

BMI readings of 25 or over should also be a warning that, unless you change your eating and lifestyle habits, you are likely to be heading for more troubled waters as you grow older.

| BMI Height (ins) | 36 | 37 | 38 | 39 | 40 | 41 | 42 | 43 | 44 | 45 | 46 | 47 | 48 | 49 | 50 | 51 | 52 | 53 | 54 |
|---|---|---|---|---|---|---|---|---|---|---|---|---|---|---|---|---|---|---|---|
| | Body Weight (lb) | | | | | | | | | | | | | | | | | | |
| 58 | 172 | 177 | 181 | 186 | 191 | 196 | 201 | 205 | 210 | 215 | 220 | 224 | 229 | 234 | 239 | 244 | 248 | 253 | 258 |
| 59 | 178 | 183 | 188 | 193 | 198 | 203 | 208 | 212 | 217 | 222 | 227 | 232 | 237 | 242 | 247 | 252 | 257 | 262 | 267 |
| 60 | 184 | 189 | 194 | 199 | 204 | 209 | 215 | 220 | 225 | 230 | 235 | 240 | 245 | 250 | 255 | 261 | 266 | 271 | 276 |
| 61 | 190 | 195 | 201 | 206 | 211 | 217 | 222 | 227 | 232 | 238 | 243 | 248 | 254 | 259 | 264 | 269 | 275 | 280 | 285 |
| 62 | 196 | 202 | 207 | 213 | 218 | 224 | 229 | 235 | 240 | 246 | 251 | 256 | 262 | 267 | 273 | 278 | 284 | 289 | 295 |
| 63 | 203 | 208 | 214 | 220 | 225 | 231 | 237 | 242 | 248 | 254 | 259 | 265 | 270 | 278 | 282 | 287 | 293 | 299 | 304 |
| 64 | 209 | 215 | 221 | 227 | 232 | 238 | 244 | 250 | 256 | 262 | 267 | 273 | 279 | 285 | 291 | 296 | 302 | 308 | 314 |
| 65 | 216 | 222 | 228 | 234 | 240 | 246 | 252 | 258 | 264 | 270 | 276 | 282 | 288 | 294 | 300 | 306 | 312 | 318 | 324 |
| 66 | 223 | 229 | 235 | 241 | 247 | 253 | 260 | 266 | 272 | 278 | 284 | 291 | 297 | 303 | 309 | 315 | 322 | 328 | 334 |
| 67 | 230 | 236 | 242 | 249 | 255 | 261 | 268 | 274 | 280 | 287 | 293 | 299 | 306 | 312 | 319 | 325 | 331 | 338 | 344 |
| 68 | 236 | 243 | 249 | 256 | 262 | 269 | 276 | 282 | 289 | 295 | 302 | 308 | 315 | 322 | 328 | 335 | 341 | 348 | 354 |
| 69 | 243 | 250 | 257 | 263 | 270 | 277 | 284 | 291 | 297 | 304 | 311 | 318 | 324 | 331 | 338 | 345 | 351 | 358 | 365 |
| 70 | 250 | 257 | 264 | 271 | 278 | 285 | 292 | 299 | 306 | 313 | 320 | 327 | 334 | 341 | 348 | 355 | 362 | 369 | 376 |
| 71 | 257 | 265 | 272 | 279 | 286 | 293 | 301 | 308 | 315 | 322 | 329 | 338 | 343 | 351 | 358 | 365 | 372 | 379 | 386 |
| 72 | 265 | 272 | 279 | 287 | 294 | 302 | 309 | 316 | 324 | 331 | 338 | 346 | 353 | 361 | 368 | 375 | 383 | 390 | 397 |
| 73 | 272 | 280 | 288 | 295 | 302 | 310 | 318 | 325 | 333 | 340 | 348 | 355 | 363 | 371 | 378 | 386 | 393 | 401 | 408 |
| 74 | 280 | 287 | 295 | 303 | 311 | 319 | 326 | 334 | 342 | 350 | 358 | 365 | 373 | 381 | 389 | 396 | 404 | 412 | 420 |
| 75 | 287 | 295 | 303 | 311 | 319 | 327 | 335 | 343 | 351 | 359 | 367 | 375 | 383 | 391 | 399 | 407 | 415 | 423 | 431 |
| 76 | 295 | 304 | 312 | 320 | 328 | 336 | 344 | 353 | 361 | 369 | 377 | 385 | 394 | 402 | 410 | 418 | 426 | 435 | 443 |

### BMI in Action

A thin, active 17-year old lad will probably have a BMI of seven.

A slim and reasonably active adult may have fat totalling around fifteen.

If you're getting on in years and spend your life typing and editing, your body mass may be around twenty-nine. This is the top end of the overweight area and heading for the obese area.

If you're a real telly-tubby, your body mass may be forty-five. This is life threatening even if you don't have diabetes. See your doctor about it right away.

### Shape

Pear-shaped weight that sits on your thighs isn't as harmful as apple-shaped weight that hangs around the middle, because the fat on the outside is only half the story. The fat on the inside is wrapped around and marbled through the organs. Fat isn't inert. It doesn't sit there doing nothing. It produces chemicals and even some hormones, which may add to your problems.

### Age

Every leaflet and book on dieting or diabetes shows similar BMI tables but they don't account for age. The metabolism slows down as we age, and relatively slim people thicken (physically!) a little with age. One book that I've come across uses a complex formula that does account for age, and this gives a lot more leeway for an older person. This makes sense, as oldies can't run around all day long.

A full hysterectomy can add two-and-a-half stones, and giving up smoking can add another two or three stones. Thus, if you're a female ex-smoker in your mid-sixties who has had a full hysterectomy (e.g. including removing the ovaries) and who has pre-diabetes or type 2 diabetes, you can expect to be overweight. Having said that, you can add ten years to your life by losing the excess flab, so it's really worth making the effort. I have exactly these problems myself, so I sympathise with you.

# 13

# Other Health Situations

*High Blood Pressure ~ Cholesterol ~ Contraceptive Pills and Devices ~ Pregnancy ~ Gestational Diabetes ~*

*The waiters' eyes sparkled and their pencils flew as she proceeded to eviscerate my wallet - pate, Whitstable oysters, a sole, filet mignon, and a favourite salad of the Nizam of Hyderabad, made of shredded five-pound notes.*
S. J. Perelman

Diabetics often have health problems in addition to their diabetes; typically high blood pressure, high cholesterol and being overweight.

## High Blood Pressure

Sodium chloride is common table salt and this is no good for high blood pressure. You can buy an alternative salt based on potassium chloride, called "Lo Salt", but I haven't come across any dieticians recommending it.

When you're doing the cooking, you might still want to put a little salt into boiled potatoes and pasta, because these foods taste like boiled socks without it, but other boiled vegetables work perfectly well without salt, and even sweet-corn tastes fine without it. You may actually notice an improvement in taste, because you'll start to taste the food itself rather than the salt. If you're cooking for a family or friends, put a couple of saltcellars on the table, so those who love salt can add it to their meal.

## Cholesterol

This is a serious problem that requires much more help and advice than I can give you in this book, but here are some basic ideas to keep you going until you can buy books on the subject, or until you can ask for specialist help.

*Things to restrict or avoid:*
~ Eat meats such as beef, lamb and pork no more than three times a week.
~ Only eat processed and deli meats such as salami on rare occasions.
~ Avoid pâté, because its main constituent is fat.
~ Avoid lard, goose and beef dripping and butter.
~ Avoid trans fats (hydrogenated fat or oil).
~ Avoid cream or full cream milk.
~ Avoid Indian takeaways cooked in ghee (melted butter).

*Here are healthier options:*
~ Choose spreads over butter, but avoid those that contain a lot of trans fat or hydrogenated fat.
~ Beans lower cholesterol and there are 50 different kinds. These can be fresh, dried, canned or frozen.
~ Choose sunflower, rapeseed or olive oil to cook with.
~ Use olive oil as a dressing for salads, marinades and so on.
~ Drink semi-skimmed milk, and use skimmed milk in cooking.
~ Choose tandoori and tikka takeaways with boiled rice and vegetables.
~ Eat eggs, but within reasonable limits.
~ Eat lots of fresh, smoked or canned fish.
~ Eat an occasional fish and chip meal from the chippy, but remove some of the batter.

~ Eat vegetables, green-leaf foods, salad and fruit. Fruit and veg can be fresh, canned, frozen or dried.
~ Eat brown or brownish breads and seeded breads.

### Contraceptive Pills and Devices
There doesn't seem to be a problem with any contraceptive pill or device, but you must ask your health advisor about this.

### Pregnancy
If you're a diabetic and you want to get pregnant, or if you find yourself pregnant, get advice as soon as possible and get as much monitoring as is necessary throughout the pregnancy. Pregnancy puts extra strain on the body, but with care and with medical help, you should be able to have at least one child. You may actually end up fitter than non-diabetic women, due to the care that you have to take. Aim to have a 4-7 mmol/l average blood glucose level at all times. You will have the baby in hospital, possibly in a large hospital where they have more staff and facilities. You can breast feed your baby.

Enlist as much help after the baby is born as possible, and get your partner to help out. Having a baby is knackering, even for a non-diabetic, and the disturbed nights after what is, in effect, an operation, are very fatiguing. Let the housework go, or get a cleaner in to help you, and rest whenever the baby rests. If you have an older child already, don't farm it out to relatives for long periods at a time, or it will feel unwanted and it will never get over that feeling. Let a variety of relatives and friends take the child for an afternoon here and there, and make it sound like a treat, rather than a means of shuffling it off so that you can have a rest.

Apparently, breastfeeding may help to prevent your own child from becoming diabetic. It could be worth checking among your diabetic friends and relatives as to whether they were breastfed or not, as that might be an interesting bit of research.

Take your partner to the clinic and give him the books on diabetes to read, because he will need to know the symptoms of a potentially dangerous hypo (typically, funny breathing and tossing around in bed while asleep). Keep glucose pills in the drawer by the bed. He must know how to administer insulin if you're on injections. Educate your partner and include him in everything. Men are very good at the complexities of life with a diabetic partner, because so much of diabetes is a techie problem and they are designed to deal with such things.

It is worth bearing in mind that diabetes increases the risk of stillbirth, infant death and a baby being born with serious abnormalities, so if you are not absolutely devoted to the idea of having children or prepared to take your chances, perhaps avoid getting pregnant at all.

### *Gestational Diabetes*

Gestational diabetes comes on in pregnancy but normally disappears again after the birth. The causes are unclear, and the pressures that a pregnancy puts on the body might be part of the story. However, it also looks as though in some cases, a hormone in the placenta tells the glands in the pancreas to produce less insulin. God only knows why this is, as it can only cause trouble, and the pregnant woman may have to take pills or even inject with insulin during the pregnancy. Once the baby (and more to the point, the placenta) is delivered, the disease starts to subside. Sometimes, this is an indication that the person will develop type 2 diabetes later in life, but sometimes it's just one of those things.

One problem that you must watch out for is the lack of knowledge, and even a lack of interest in diabetes within the medical profession. If you are not normally diabetic, but you become so when pregnant, ask your GP to refer you to a diabetes clinic for the duration of the pregnancy and above all, educate yourself about diabetes via books like this and perhaps join "Diabetes UK" to get up-to-date information.

# 14

# Are You Overweight?

*Sodit! ~ Skipping Meals ~ Weight Loss: the Male Method ~ Weight Loss: the Woman's Way ~ Answers and Measurements ~ Some thoughts on the Subject of Weight ~ Survivors ~ Useful Tips ~ Surgery as an Option ~ Benefits ~ Let them eat Cake! ~ Sasha's Cake Recipe ~ Finally*

> *Ask not what you can do for your country;*
> *Ask what's for lunch.*

Orson Welles

Type 2 diabetes itself tends to make the sufferer fat, and the medication puts on even more weight, so it's hard for the diabetic to win the weight battle. Nevertheless, every kilo lost is a kilo on the road to health.

~ Until you lose the excess weight and get your diabetes under control, only eat products that contain less than 6 grams of sugar per 100g.
~ Even when you're fine, keep the sugar content of processed foods down as far as possible.
~ Take a walk or do some other kind of exercise every day.
~ Join a slimming club, either in person or online.
~ Buy magazines on slimming for ideas and inspiration.

If you haven't had diabetes for long or if you're pre-diabetic, you will still have some beta cells spewing out insulin. In this case, losing weight will help clear fat from your liver and other organs and allow them to take up the insulin and work properly. If you have been suffering from diabetes for years, losing weight may not do much good, if your pancreas is damaged. However, losing weight will improve your general health and that will help you cope with your diabetes better.

Write down everything that you eat for three days, as you will then see what you're actually consuming.

Make a shopping list and *use it*

### *Sodit!*

If you do eat something wrong, don't say, "Sodit! I've broken my diet, now I might as well eat the whole block of cheese or the rest of the family-size chocolate cake". A dieter who goes OTT will just feel nauseous, depressed, guilty and fat, but a diabetic will be sacrificing his eyes, kidneys, legs and life - for the sake of a pizza, a cheese or a creamy dessert. Don't go the "Sodit!" route.

### *Skipping Meals*

All diets include three meals a day and a couple of snacks - and that is even for those who don't have diabetes. We must eat several times a day and never skip meals. Little and often is the best way.

I've discovered that Tesco's Internet slimming club has a programme for diabetics, so that's worth checking out.So does Slimming World, and I'm sure that other similar organisations do, too.

### *Weight loss: The Male Method*

Men tend to think that the way to lose weight is to join a gym. In reality, they pay the joining fee and then go once out of curiosity and once more out of determination. They mean to go on a regular basis thereafter, but they are actually far too busy to get around to it.

When you think about it, gyms probably couldn't operate successfully if all the people who paid joining fees actually attended! Quite likely, it's the hefty donations given by the charitable members who don't actually attend regularly that keep gyms viable. There are some vain or fanatical men who spend all their spare time pumping things at a gym, but before I would consider choosing one as a life partner, I would want him to get his brains tested...

Some men think that cutting down from ten beers a night to eight will do the trick. Cutting down from ten beers a night to two is a better choice, as it will do wonders for the blood glucose as well as dramatically reduce the calorie intake.

## *Weight loss: The Woman's Way*

The woman's method is to read about a diet in a magazine and then try it. Four days later, she gets on her scales hoping that the five stone she needs to lose has magic'd itself away. After all, she has been bloody hungry for half a week, so she deserves to be a least a couple of stone lighter. To her chagrin, she sees that she has lost about a half pound - if that. She decides to leave it for a while. Several months later, she tries another magazine diet with the same lack of result. She then buys some (sugar-filled) shakes and tries them. Then she tries the bowl of delicious (sugar-filled) breakfast cereal for breakfast and lunch method. She manages to survive on this for a day - but by the second day, she is so hungry that she could eat a telephone directory! At this point, she says, "I've tried every diet going and nothing works for me".

## *Some Thoughts on the Subject of Weight*

While researching this book, I watched a TV programme about a bunch of extremely overweight teenagers. The participants hoped, and sincerely believed, that their weight would fall off almost within hours of starting a planned walk. In the event, after a week of walking, they lost very little weight, and one or two of them put weight on! The self-indulgent youngsters groused and complained non-stop, while the laid-back physiotherapist who walked with them just kept quiet. However, on one occasion, while watching them go through several bags of chips each, he commented out of sheer frustration, "You really do eat a tremendous amount of crap!" The message here is that, while exercise is good for all round fitness, it won't take weight off while you still eat the wrong food.

### Survivors

Some people can hang on to weight in any circumstances. I've known two concentration camp victims who survived the holocaust because they had a natural tendency to obesity. One woman spent two years in a German concentration camp, and when she came out, she was a size 14! If Hitler couldn't make fat people thin, what chance do we have? Of course, these examples are no doubt exceptions, but it's nice to find possible reasons why one isn't losing weight as one should...

### Useful Tips

*These tips might help:*
*Shopping*
~ Make a shopping list, as this cuts down impulse buying.
~ Never shop on an empty stomach (this tip is also a good money saver!).
~ If you have to visit the aisles that sell cakes, biscuits and sweets because you're buying for others, shop quickly and then move away.
~ Park away from the supermarket entrance, so that you have further to walk.
*Other*
~ Don't fry if you can cook some other way, such as grilling bacon or baking oven chips. Incidentally, I recently saw a TV programme featuring a woman who needed to lose weight, and she admitted that she fried everything, including oven chips!

~ We all fry things occasionally, so buy a very good pan that doesn't stick; then smear it with a little oil, or spray it with a little special low-fat stuff.

~ If you were brought up to eat everything on your plate, ignore this programming and break the pattern.

~ Nuts are fattening, but sometimes a few nuts make a good snack.

~ Bake a potato in the microwave and eat that with a salad.

~ Eat food that weighs a lot, such as soup, salads, potatoes, sweet potatoes, vegetables, rice, beans and granary bread as this will fill you up.

~ Eat five portions of fruit or vegetables a day.

~ Always eat breakfast.

~ Eat a variety of foods.

~ Sit at a table and eat in a civilised manner, using proper cutlery.

~ Put your knife and fork down between mouthfuls, and pick them up again when your mouth is empty.

~ It takes a while for the stomach to register that it's filling up, so you need to give it time to do this. The way to make this happen is to eat slowly.

~ Take a walk every day, if you can.

~ Walk up and down stairs rather than taking the lift.

### Surgery as an Option

I'm sure every dietician on earth would argue against liposuction or surgery as an answer to weighty problems, but I think the time will come when stomach bands and bypasses become commonplace. I read an article about this in which the surgeon said, "For some people, it's the only way, because for them, diet, exercises and lifestyle changes won't cut it."

I don't know enough about these procedures to recommend them, but I do know that if I were 30 stone and gaining more each day, I'd sell my car, raise the money and say goodbye to my stomach!

### Benefits

Lose a bit of weight and your skin will look better, you will be livelier and you will have more strength and stamina than people half your age have.

### Let Them Eat Cake!

Diabetes encourages you to cook and to experiment with recipes. My attempts at brown flour pastry were a good laugh. It turned out so hard and tough that my daughter asked me to make a piece measuring 18" x 18" specially for her so that she could use it to mend her garden shed!

I recently adapted a recipe to make a great low sugar, low fat and high fibre cake, and it was a success. It might need a bit more tweaking, but if you try it once or twice, you will come up with your own variation on a theme.

**I suggest adding a little cinnamon in the following recipe, as it goes with apple and more to the point, it's supposed to stimulate the production of insulin.**

## Sasha's Cake Recipe

| | |
|---|---|
| 100ml | No-added-sugar orange juice. |
| | *(No-added-sugar apple or any other juice would do).* |
| 100g | Mixed dried fruit. |
| | *Raisins, currants or anything of the kind will work.* |
| 100g | Spread. |
| | *Find one that suits you best.* |
| 3 | Large eggs. |
| 300g | Crusty, wholemeal bread flour. |
| 50g | Fruisana, or similar fruit sugar. |
| 2 tsps | Splenda powder. |
| 1 tsp | *(level tsps)* Baking powder. |
| 2 | small apples. |
| | *Peel, core and cut up into small pieces.* |
| 1/2 tsp | *(level tsp)* cinnamon. |
| | *(Perhaps try one cake without cinnamon, and the next with it, to see which you prefer).* |

## Method

Preheat an oven to 180C/350F or gas 4.

Grease a seven- or eight-inch cake tin.

Warm the juice and dried fruit in a saucepan. Don't let it boil.

Cream the spread, sugar and sweetener with a wooden spoon.

Put in a teaspoon of flour and add an egg. Cream the egg.

Repeat with the other two eggs (a bit of flour and then the egg).

Beat well.

Mix the flour and baking powder.

Fold-in half of the flour.

Add the dried fruit and juice.

Add the apple pieces.

Fold-in the rest of the flour.

Put into the cake tin and bake for 40 minutes.

Cool, cut into pieces.


Then, move out of the way quickly, or you'll be killed in the rush!

# 15

# Children

*School ~ Teens ~ Will your Child get Diabetes?*

> *Your body is the baggage you must carry though life.*
> *The more excess baggage, the shorter the trip.*

E. Glasgow

I haven't specifically gone into the problems of diabetic children in this book. The chances are that the child will be type 1, so he or she will need to inject insulin. There should be plenty of professional help on hand, but you should join Diabetes UK (www.diabetes.org.uk), and also find out all you can about the management of a diabetic child. You must also buy a box file and keep all relevant information in it.

## *School*

If your child is young, write to his or her school head and relevant teachers about your child's condition, and keep a copy of the letters in your home file. Explain that the child may need to use the loo more frequently than others. If the youngster feels funny due to hunger, or if he or she knows that a game of football or a gym session is coming up, he or she may need to take a biscuit from a pocket or bag and eat it discreetly. Explain why this is and why the child shouldn't be punished.

Some teachers are wonderful, but others are uninterested, unsympathetic, unhelpful and thick. Teachers have favourites, and a child that requires extra effort is unlikely to qualify as a favourite. Keep on plugging away politely until the teacher gets the message. Where older children are concerned, they will probably be capable of dealing with their condition for themselves, but if they happen to be cursed with a dense or unsympathetic teacher, you might need to go to the school and have a quiet word. Never steam in to a school in a temper. Treat all teachers and other officials as if you are a salesman and the official is a valued customer. Be very pleasant, speak in a quiet, calm but firm voice and flatter them. This may make you feel like a cheese-eating surrender-monkey, but this book is about survival in the real world, so if a bit of flattery is going to grease the gears for your child, do it.

(I gather that a rather nasty tradition that didn't exist in my children's day now exists. I understand that it is now obligatory to give a teacher a Christmas present, and I hear tales that the best gift-giver's children tend to receive the best treatment from some teachers. Therefore, if it is now necessary to bribe such people, why not bribe them with copies of this book? Perhaps I can bring out a gold-plated edition for this purpose!).

Ensure that your child or your teenager measures his or her blood glucose before doing heavy-duty activity. The blood glucose must be over 4mmol/l. If it isn't, then the kid must eat a couple of biscuits and a banana to avoid a possible hypo.

## Teens

If your teens go out for the evening, they will yak with their friends, drink and dance or leap around, but they won't have a meal. Their blood glucose will be sliding down the scale by the time they come home, so leave a snack or sandwich out for them to eat before going to bed to avoid the killer nocturnal hypo.

Whether the teen is diabetic or not, if they do drink, then leave the "Trinity" out for them so that they can grab it when they eventually crawl out of bed. The "Trinity" is water, fruit juice or tomato juice and two Paracetamol tablets. Jan suggests Eno's Fruit Salts before bed, and Alka Seltzer is another well-known option.

If a teen falls for someone, and the object of their love laughs at them for being diabetic or for having bruises or lumps from the insulin injections, the teen must dump this rotten person immediately. Illness isn't something to laugh at. Two good sayings that you can pass onto you youngster are: "Time wounds all heels" and "God pays debts without money." In short, nasty people always do get their comeuppance, although unfortunately, we aren't always around to see it.

### Will Your Child Get Diabetes?

Possibly. The chance of a child with two diabetic parents getting the disease is said to be 40 per cent, but even twins whose parents are both diabetic don't always both get it. My first husband developed type 2 diabetes when he was in his sixties, so my children have two diabetic parents. So far, they're both fine.

The good news is that new treatments are coming along all the time, and by the time your children are grown up, there should be a cure. At the moment, all you can do is to attend to their diet and get them to take some exercise.

# 16

# Medicines and Medical People

---

*Pre-diabetic ~ Type 2 Diabetes ~ Type 1 Diabetes ~ Both Types ~Unhelpful Help ~ Pharmacists Can Help*

> *Medicine is the only profession that labours incessantly to destroy the reason for its own existence*

James Bryce

This is a guide to everyday living rather than a medical book as such, so I urge you to get all the advice you can, and to read other books on the subject of diabetes. However, here is a brief overview of the medicine scene, and what you can do to help yourself.

## Pre-diabetic

You may get away with careful eating and exercise, but you should get annual blood and eye tests, and use a home blood tester occasionally to ensure that your diabetes isn't climbing into the type 2 range.

Don't ignore your condition, because a teaspoonful of self-help at this stage can save you many tears and much disablement later in life.

## Type 2 Diabetes

You may be prescribed pills to stimulate your pancreas into making more insulin. In some cases, this is the right treatment, but it can work the pancreas so hard that it loses what ability it still has. Another kind of drug will stimulate your liver into doing something useful with the insulin that you do make. Ensure that you know what you're taking, what it's supposed to do for you and what side effects there may be. If you get side effects, go straight back to the doctor so that you can switch to some other pill. If the pills make you hypoglycaemic, you may need to lower the dose or change to something else. If you don't get enough help or information from your GP, ask to be referred to a diabetes clinic.

Buy a date pillbox that has little compartments marked Monday, Tuesday, Wednesday, etc. and put a week's supply of pills in it. That way, you won't forget to take them or overdose by taking them twice in one day.

If you're told you need to inject insulin for a while, don't get upset. Insulin injections can give your pancreas a much-needed rest.

## Type 1 Diabetes

Get help. Become knowledgeable. Take control of your condition and your life. Knowledge is the key to survival.

## Unhelpful Help

If you don't get enough help from the National Health Service, buy books, search the 'Net and find out all you can about your condition. Join Diabetes UK (www.diabetes.org.uk). Buy a blood test machine and use it occasionally, until you know what pushes your blood glucose up.

If a doctor or nurse is unsympathetic, it's probably because they don't know much about diabetes. Everybody has heard of diabetes, but the fact is that it's a very specialised area of medicine. If someone shouts at you or blames you for making yourself ill (say, because the doctor or nurse decides that you have been eating the wrong things or getting drunk), insist on seeing someone else.

If you travel a lot, you may wish to get a letter from your doctor to carry around with you. This could well be a useful tip anyway, in case someone needs guidance in assisting you.

There are good health centres and lousy ones everywhere, and there are pleasant and knowledgeable medical staff and dreadful ones everywhere. The one person you can definitely rely on is yourself, so learn all you can about diabetes and keep up with modern developments at all times.

Not every diabetic is the same, so what suits your relative, friend or neighbour may not suit you. You will react to food, alcohol, exercise and drugs differently to them. Each diabetic is an individual, which is why it is so important for you to become your own doctor.

### *Pharmacists Can Help*

If you or someone you care for use the same medicines regularly, you may be able to benefit from repeat dispensing from the pharmacist. This means you won't need to visit the surgery to see the doctor or practice nurse every time you need more medicine. Talk to the pharmacist about this service. If you pay for prescriptions a pre-payment certificate will save you money. You may qualify for free prescriptions under a low-income scheme or as a diabetic. Pharmacists are often very clued up about illness and it's a good idea to ask your pharmacist for advice on minor or everyday matters.

Some pharmacists in the UK are able to offer blood tests and other help that will save you from having to visit your GP quite that often.

# 17

# Being Active

*Activity ~Type 1 Diabetics ~ Non-Severe Type 2 Diabetes ~ Shoes ~ Hunger and Weight ~ Tai Chi*

> *Never eat more than you can lift.*
>
> Miss Piggy

### Activity

Being active means everything from a stroll around the shops to climbing Everest. The level of activity must be judged against the level of diabetes. In some cases, this needs careful assessment and management, especially in the case of insulin dependent diabetes of either type.

Activity releases "feel good" endomorphic hormones that will cheer you up.

You should wear one of those "medical" bracelets or necklace pendants when you go out and do strenuous things, or even when you're away on business. There are many different kinds in chemist shops and on the Internet, and some are cheap and cheerful, while others are expensive and decorative. Also keep a note in your wallet or purse, or some other relatively visible place, to show whether you're diet-controlled or on medication and what medication you are on.

Send for information to The Diabetes Exercise and Sports Association, P.O. Box 1935, Litchfield Park, AZ85340, USA. Check out www.diabetes.exercise.org

### *Type 1 Diabetes*

So far, I've not suggested anything in this book that would harm a type 1 diabetic, but when we come to the subject of sports and activities, the situation changes. It's probable that a stroll around the park, doing a salsa class once a week, playing pitch-and-putt with the kids, or going for a weekly swim will be fine. Even then, you may need to test your blood before and after exercise. If you're going to do something that puts a lot of strain on your body, or something that demands endurance, such as hiking, you need specialist advice. If you intend to be alone or to be with people who don't know about your condition and who don't know how to help you if you become ill, you really need to think again.

If your glucose level falls too low, you will have a "hypo" and it will affect your brain. You will appear drunk or weird, and even if there is someone around who knows about diabetes and who knows what to do, you will refuse help or deny that you're "hypo". You might collapse immediately or you might struggle on, fall asleep and never wake up again. Those around you need to know about your condition, and you must tell them what to look out for, and what they should do to help you. You must carry your insulin works, blood tester, glucose tablets, biscuits and orange juice or coca cola in your backpack. Keep all this and water in your car (not in the boot) when you go on trips as well. A sugar boost is a short-term solution, so the next step will be to go in search of a sandwich or a meal.

To be quite frank - if you're a type 1 diabetic or a seriously ill type 2 diabetic, you will need much more advice than I've suggested here. Read the books that I've listed in the bibliography and ask your health specialist for advice before going in for any kind of sport.

## *Non-Severe Type 2 Diabetes*

For you, exercise and maybe losing some weight will help your body get going again, and if you can get fit, you may be able to downgrade from insulin injections to pills or go from pills to diet-control. Even so, I suggest that you take care with extreme sports, seeking out medical advice before embarking on them. Tell your team members about your condition and ask them to keep an eye on you. Take your blood tester, water, pills, glucose, a sandwich and a can of "full-fat" Coke with you. Even a slog round a supermarket can make you feel ill if you do it on an empty stomach, so go shopping after you've eaten something.

Most people who have type 2 diabetes are not so much addicted to extreme sports as they are to lolling in front of the telly or the computer screen. (Don't I know it!) You must get moving. Perhaps you can teach your children to play rounders in the park, or join them in ice-skating, roller-skating or swimming. Your local adult education institute will offer classes in tap dancing, tai chi, movement for older people, salsa dancing, aerobics and many other things. Take a Frisbee, borrow some children or a dog from your neighbour and take them to the park, so that you use up some calories while you're running around and laughing. Take your boyfriend or partner to the beach and fly kites. Make a complete ass of yourself at the pitch-and-put course for an hour or so. Give it all a try. Go out, make new friends and have fun. Have a swim or go for a walk in the country. Moving around helps keep boredom and depression at bay and in an odd way, it can make you feel less hungry. Boredom makes you look for something to eat, so keep busy. Even going to the pub with friends is better than sitting around on your own.

## *Shoes*

Buy the right shoes for your sport, and ensure that they don't cut or rub your feet. If your nerve endings are damaged, you may not feel a blister forming, and it could turn into something much worse.

When shoes get old, they can fall apart inside while still looking ok on the outside, so check your shoes inside and out. Always wash and inspect your feet after exercise.

## Hunger and Weight

Exercise may give you an appetite and you might even put on a little weight if you exercise a lot. This is because you're building up muscle in place of fat. As long as your blood glucose is fine, don't worry too much about this. Remember, some diabetes drugs put weight on, but never skip injections or drugs for the sake of looking thin. Your life is more important than trying to look like a ferret faced ghost, a la Posh Beckham.

## Tai Chi

Some surveys have discovered that an hour's Tai Chi three times a week gives good results. This is a gentle exercise that calms the mind and tones the body without being harsh or hard to do. Apparently, some heavy-duty types of exercise can actually increase blood sugar levels temporarily while the body signals a need for extra glucose, but Tai Chi doesn't, so all in all, Tai Chi looks like a good thing for a diabetic person to take up.

# 18

# Breakfast

*Porridge ~ Cereals ~ Other Ideas ~ Bacon and other Meats ~ Continental Breakfast ~ Crumpets and Bagels ~ Other Breakfasts*

> *Eat breakfast like a king,*
> *lunch like a prince and dinner like a pauper.*

Adelle Davis

From now on, you must always eat breakfast. Slim people eat breakfast while overweight people don't, and then they get hungry and reach for cakes, chocolate or biscuits. You can't do that if you're diabetic.

## Porridge

If you like porridge, it fills you up and keeps you full for quite a long time. Being made from oats, it has a lower GI than other cereals. The best porridge to buy is the cheapo stuff packed in an unattractive polythene bag. The porridge in fancy cardboard packs doesn't break down in the saucepan as well, it tastes slightly dusty and it's stupidly expensive.

*This is How to Make Porridge*
~ 50g porridge oats per person
~ 300ml water per person

Put the water in a saucepan and chuck in the porridge. Bring it to the boil and stir it with a wooden spoon, then simmer it for three minutes, giving it an occasional stir.

Serve on its own, or with some semi-skimmed milk poured on top, and perhaps with sweetener or a small sprinkling of fruit sugar. You could add a little fresh or dried fruit to your porridge. Try various ways until you find what works for you.

> **Put the measuring jug, scales, saucepan and pack of porridge out the night before, so that you can make it on autopilot while dressing and getting the kids ready.**

## Cereals

Cereal with semi-skimmed milk is nice, but you should avoid children's cereals that have loads of sugar added. Old fashioned cereals, such as Cornflakes and Rice Crispies are all right, but they do have sugar in them, even though they don't have extra sugar sprinkled on top. The Special K sold as a slimming food contains a lot of sugar, so avoid that one.

Check the contents before buying anything, though, and if it has much more than 6g of sugar per 100g, find another brand.

*Cereals that appear to contain no sugar at all are:*

~ Puffed Wheat.
~ Shredded Wheat.
~ Wheatabix.
~ Oatabix.
~ Shreddies (with fruit in them, if your blood glucose level is all right, otherwise stick to the plain variety).

## Other Ideas

~ Toast with a thin scraping of jam (ordinary jam is fine).
~ Brown bread and cheese.

~ Brown toast and peanut butter (watch for trans fats, though).
~ Plain yoghurt with fresh fruit tossed into it.
~ Grapefruit is good, but it needs a lot of sweetener on it to make it edible, so a half-orange is often a better choice. It also "argues" with cholesterol medication.
~ Any fruit with yoghurt, fromàge frais or with a slice of bread.
~ Eggs.

> **Apparently recent research has shown that black tea (e.g. tea without milk added) can help combat diabetes.**

### Bacon and Other Meats
Cut some of the fat off these items and grill them.

### Continental Breakfast
This is the worst of all options, because croissants contain sugar, as do some rolls, and the rolls are usually made of high GI white flour. Try brown rolls or toasted granary bread and a smear of ordinary marmalade or jam.

> **Fizzy drinks like diet colas contain caffeine and raise blood glucose levels. Try diluted fruit juice instead.**

### Crumpets and Bagels
Look around for brown bagels or eat the (very) occasional white one for a change. Take care not to put too much spread on them, though. Crumpets make a nice change.

### Other Breakfasts
Depending upon your background, you may like cheese, cold meats, olives, pickled or salted herrings, kippers, smoked salmon or a million other things for breakfast. All these things are just fine with brown bread and a cup of fresh hot tea or decaff coffee. Caffeine raises blood glucose levels.

# 19

# Main Meals

---

*Top Tips ~ Starters and Main Courses ~ Vegetables ~
Desserts ~ Fruit and Juice ~ Cakes and Biscuits*

> *I would like to find a stew that will give me heartburn
> immediately, instead of at three o'clock in the morning.*

John Barrymore

## Top Tips

~ Eat a varied diet and try new things from time to time to avoid getting stale and bored.

~ Eat lots of vegetables, salad and fruit.

~ Almost anything that you cook yourself for starters and main courses will be fine.

## Starters and Main Courses

Any starter will work, although pâté is fattening. Homemade soup is a great filler and it costs very little to make or buy. Any normal kind of food is fine, so choose meat, fish, smoked fish, shellfish, eggs, cheese, veggies, salad and anything else in between. It's better to eat the wrong thing on occasion than to limit yourself to a few types of food.

Gravy granules, Oxo cubes and similar things are salty, so if you have high blood pressure, don't use these things too often.

Keep an eye on shop-bought sauces such as sweet and sour sauce, and things in packets. You must check the sugar content before buying these items. Until you're stabilised, stick to 6g of sugar per 100g. If you buy ready-cooked foods in cans, packets, pots or any other container, check the contents for sugar, and perhaps also for salt and fat. Some ready meals are loaded with these things to stop them from being tasteless. Many contain white flour or cornstarch, and they may contain preservatives and colour as well. Use packet foods, pizzas and stuff like that very sparingly.

Basmati rice has a low GI but it's dry, so you might want to use stock (a little soup makes a good quick stock) or gravy with it. Apparently the partly cooked types of long grain rice have a lower GI than standard long grain rice. If you only like bog-standard Uncle Ben's rice, that's fine as long as you don't eat it too often. Starchy foods, such as potatoes, rice, pasta and grains are good with meat, vegetables, gravy, salad and other things, as these slow down their GI. When you buy canned foods, such as peas or baked beans, choose those without added sugar. If you have blood pressure problems, use Lo Salt. Try cooking with herbs, pepper or lemon to give flavour.

All fish is great, as it's low GI, low calorie and some fish contain omega 3 and omega 6, both of which are beneficial. The downside with fish is that it becomes higher on the Glycaemic Index and higher in calories when coated with breadcrumbs or batter and fried. Crumbed and grilled fish, as in fish fingers, is a better option.

***Here are a few stray tips that I have come across in my research:***

~ Vinegar lowers the GI when added to foods, so if you like it, sprinkle some on your fish and chips.
~ Shellfish contains some cholesterol, but this doesn't have much effect on blood cholesterol, and it is low in fat, so it makes a nice change.

~ Surprisingly, sausages and bacon are medium GI.

~ Swedes, carrots and parsnips are high GI, but they also contain fibre, and this is good for a diabetic, so don't avoid them, but put some green veggies or meat with them to slow down their absorption.

~ If you buy a curry, add some cooked vegetables and potatoes to the mixture, this will lower the calories and make it more balanced.

~ Add extra veggies to a pizza to make it more balanced.

~ Make your own lasagna with added veggies.

~ Oven chips are lower in fat than fried chips.

~ Yams or sweet potatoes are low GI, as are ordinary new potatoes.

## *Vegetables*

There's a school of thought that boiling vegetables and throwing away the water that they are cooked in wastes their goodness. If you're worried about this, you could try steaming or microwaving your veggies. Some vegetables work in the microwave - frozen peas are okay, for example, but other things (sprouts, cabbage) are revolting when steamed or nuked. Make home-cooked soup occasionally, as that's a way of getting the goodness from a variety of vegetables. Also make salads and crudités of finely chopped vegetables with dips or mayonnaise. Stir-fry veggies or salad wraps are a nice idea, too.

There is a downside to eating a lot of fruit and vegetables if you aren't used to doing so, and that is trapped wind, bloating, breaking wind and creating unsociable smells. If this bothers you, try those yoghurt drink products that you see advertised on the television, but do remember to check the sugar content in them. I have discovered Actimel and Yoplait to be within reasonable tolerances, but always check - ingredients do change sometimes.

Veggies fill you up and keep your blood glucose down, so aim to fill 1/3 to 1/2 of your plate with them.

*Desserts*

~ Tesco sells sugar-free custard powder.

~ Some yoghurts are low enough in sugar for you to eat. Try the Weight Watchers products.

~ Canned fruit in juice is all right, if you drain off the juice.

~ Fromàge frais is good with fruit.

~ Fruit sugar is all right for occasional use, especially if your blood glucose is within tolerances.

~ Try agave nectar. This is made from the Agave cactus and it tastes rather like honey but it is low GI.

~ Try making fruit pies with a mixture of white and brown (or beige) flour to reduce the GI, and use Splenda powder for cooking. Alternatively, make fruit pies or pieces of fruit and nuts, wrapped in filo pastry and baked.

~ Melon makes a great dessert. It has quite a high GI, but as it doesn't contain any carbohydrate and it does contain fibre.

~ Milk puddings, such as rice, sago, semolina and tapioca, work perfectly well with Splenda in place of sugar.

~ Weight Watchers make a very good sugar-free jelly and also an instant whip that is really delicious.

~ Walls makes a reduced sugar vanilla icecream, and Asda sells a diabetic ice cream made by Franks. This only comes in vanilla flavour, but you can dress it up with fruit pieces.

I tried a recipe for banana bread. It was quick and easy to make and, like all banana bread, it looked a little greyish in colour. It tasted very good, but you might want to add a teaspoonful of powdered sweetener to the mixture.

## Fruit and Juice

Fruit is ideal as a dessert or snack. Mix and match the type of fruit that you eat, because some fruits are more sugary than others, especially some of the tropical fruits. Fruit-juice counts as one portion of fruit, but it can be high in sugar so don't drink too much of it. You can always dilute fruit juice with water.

*Cakes and Biscuits*

Make your own cakes, either from recipes from diabetic cookery books or by reducing the amount of fat and sugar in a normal recipe by half. If you absolutely can't do without shop-bought cake, buy malt loaf or fruitcake, as they tend to be lower in fat and sugar. Frankly, I avoid all shop-bought cake, because one tiny slice just isn't enough for me and I know I will eat too much of it.

If you must have a biscuit, stick to rich tea, hobnobs, garibaldi and ginger nuts, as these are lower in sugar and fat than others. Avoid chocolate biscuits and wafer or sandwich biscuits that contain sweet creamy fillings.

# 20

# Packed Lunches and Picnics

*Sandwiches and Rolls ~ Pasta ~ Veggies ~ Desserts ~ Snacks ~ Avoid ~ Soup ~ Drinks*

> *Rice is great if you want 2,000 of something.*
Mitch Hedburg

My daughter Helen, has always made up packed lunches for her husband Riccardo and herself, so I've turned to her for ideas.

### Sandwiches and Rolls

There are many different kinds of bread. If you have a problem with white bread, there are plenty of other varieties to choose from. If you're fine with white bread, but you want to keep the bread part of the meal to a minimum, choose pita bread or tortilla wraps.

Fillings can include something that you buy, or a cut from something that you have leftover in the fridge. Helen uses salami, ham, beef, lamb and sometimes pâté, although that is high in cholesterol. She says that English, American or continental mustards are good with ham, beef or lamb. She sometimes makes a BLT (bacon, lettuce and tomato) sandwich.

Tuna with mayo is good, and smoked salmon or smoked trout are nice for a treat. Eggs can be hard-boiled and sliced, or hard-boiled and chopped with mayo. She puts a bit of lettuce in with dry meats. She doesn't put cress in egg sandwiches, because he says that it goes stringy and then tastes like dental floss, while tomatoes make the bread go soggy.

Cheese can be spread-able, hard or soft cheese. If you're on a diet or need to restrict your fat intake, choose Edam, Gouda, Brie or any light or low fat variety of cheese.

Try pita bread or a wrap with a salad and egg or salad and anchovy filling.

> *I've just come across someone who likes beetroot and corned beef sandwiches. Well... each to his own, I say.*

### Pasta

Being married to an Italian, Helen always has pasta in their house. Pasta is made from durum wheat, which is relatively good on the GI scale. She piles pasta into plastic boxes with peppers, tomato, olives, sweetcorn, tuna and mayo. Helen says to remember to put in a plastic fork and some paper napkins.

Helen says that you can use the same recipes with cooked rice or couscous. Sometimes she makes up a pot of potato salad, or perhaps Russian salad, which is potato salad with some chopped, cooked carrots, peas and onions in it. Home made pie or solid types of quiche made with brown flour pastry can be useful.

### Veggies

Carrot sticks, celery sticks and whole cherry tomatoes are good, and you can put in a whole hardboiled egg, if you like. A wedge of cheese, or a couple of those little cheeses encased in waxy stuff, are good.

### Desserts

Helen often puts in an apple, pear, banana, a few grapes, a couple of plums or a peach. She also suggests a pot of yoghurt (look for those that are low in sugar), or fromàge frais. If you make suitable cakes, put a slice of cake in as well.

### Snacks
Helen says crispbreads are not filling enough for a packed lunch, but they make good snacks, as do nuts and even a little dark chocolate on occasion.

### Avoid
Commercial pies, pasties and sausage rolls, as these contain too much white flour, cornstarch, fat and salt. Helen says that a "wrap" is better if there's no other option.

So-called healthy cereal bars are very high in sugar, but two makes, called Trek and Nakd, are low sugar (at present...) and both are on sale in health food shops.

Avoid getting hungry and then grabbing a Mars Bar out of the machine at work. If you feel a hypo coming on, eat a glucose sweet and go in search of a sandwich - even one with white bread if that's all you can find. Raisins and currants are useful as a quick hypo pickup, as are dates and figs.

### Soup
If you have a microwave or cooker at work, a can of soup is a good lunch snack. The creamy ones are higher in calories than the broth types and all commercial soups contain salt, which matters if you have high blood pressure. The "big soups" make a nutritious lunch. Some canned soups have a lot of sugar in them, so check the label before buying them.

### Drinks
In general, any sugar-free or no-added-sugar drink is fine, so sling a can or bottle into the lunch box. Riccardo is an electrician, so when he is working in a cold environment, Helen makes him a flask of coffee or a flask of home-made soup.

# 21

# Desperate Measures

*Feeling Hungry ~ Some Alternatives to Food*

*Researchers have found that chocolate produces some of the same reactions in the brain as marijuana.*
*The researchers also discovered other similarities between the two, but can't remember what they are.*
Matt Laur (on NBC's Today Show)

### Feeling Hungry

Getting hungry between meals is a problem not only for diabetics, but also for dieters and health conscious people. Try some of these ideas:

~ Drinking helps to fill you up, so if you feel hungry, try a glass of water, a no-added-sugar drink, a diet ginger beer or a cup of tea. Believe it or not, you can sometimes feel hungry when you're actually thirsty, so it's always worth trying a drink first.

~ A couple of slices of (brown) bread with marmite, a bit of ham, a piece of cheese, some fish paste or even a small scrape of ordinary jam will fill a hole. Drink tea or coffee with this and you will soon feel better.

~ Throw a potato into the microwave, and when it's cooked, toss in some spread, sugar-free baked beans, cheese or leftovers from the fridge.

~ Eat some nuts - especially almonds - as these are good for your diabetes and they are a nice treat.

~ Fruit is an obvious snack for diabetics, as are raw veggies such as carrots, celery, radish and so on.

~ Buy an exotic fruit or one you've never tried from time to time.

I know that dieticians will have a flying hissy fit at the following suggestions, but they can afford to be school-marmish, because they don't have your problems, or your hunger.

### These tips might save your sanity:

~ Potato crisps are fattening and high GI, but find ones made from actual potatoes rather than dried potato, flour, cornstarch, dried milk and so on. Weight Watchers' Hoops are very nice, and they are low in sugar and fat.

~ There are loads of cracker biscuits on the market, too. Some contain cheese or herbs. These are fattening and they contain high GI white flour, so you can't eat too many of them, but there are times when a carrot stick just isn't going to cut it!

~ I found loads of ideas in a magazine for lower calorie versions of food and alcoholic drinks, so it's worth buying health or slimming magazines from time to time, for inspiration and encouragement.

~ All books on diabetes, and every nutritionist, will tell you to avoid diabetic products, but I find the shortbread biscuits all right, though I never eat more than one biscuit a day. Sometimes, one biscuit with a cup of coffee can save you from going round the bend!

~ There are several companies that make black chocolate bars with a very high chocolate content - around 75% to 80%. These contain very little sugar and fat, but they don't taste that good!

*Some Alternatives to Food*

~ Go out for a walk.

~ Take a leisurely bath.

~ Go to the pub and meet your friends.

~ Play sports, go jogging, or dance.

~ Phone a friend.

~ Do a crossword.

~ Make love.

~ Pray for strength and try to keep a positive mental attitude.

# 22

# Dining Out and Takeaways

*Dinner Parties ~ Afternoon Tea ~ Quality Restaurants and American Style Dining ~ a Really Posh Restaurant ~ a Carvery ~ Going for an Indian ~ Chinese Nosh ~ Water ~ a Doner Dinner ~ Fish and Chips ~ a Classic Burger Meal ~ Kentucky Fried Chicken ~ Filled Potatoes ~ Pub Grub ~ Sarnies ~ a Good Italian Restaurant ~ Pizza and Pasta ~ Thank God it's Friday ~ Tapas ~ the Local Caff ~ Meals on Wheels ~ Cooked Supermarket Food ~ Drinks ~ Tea and Coffee*

> *The art of dining well is no slight art,*
> *the pleasure not a slight pleasure*

Michel de Montaigne

### Dinner Parties

If you go to someone else's house for a sit down meal, tell them that you can eat the starter and main course, but you won't bother with the dessert unless it's fruit salad, with or without cream, depending upon your cholesterol levels. Alternatively, ask your host to provide dried fruit and nuts or cheese, crackers and celery. Buffets are usually fine, as you can pick and choose without anyone being the wiser.

## *Afternoon Tea*

Afternoon tea is a nightmare. I don't mean high tea, I mean the kind of afternoon tea that consists of cakes and biscuits. Ask the host to give you suitable food, such as an egg mayonnaise sandwich on granary bread if you can. The alternative is to eat something before you go and then take a small helping of each food. One "wrong meal" won't kill you, but you should try to dilute this with a glass or two of water.

## *Quality Restaurants and American Style Dining*

Whenever I have a meal out with Americans, I am often embarrassed by the amount of fuss that they make about what they want and how they want it cooked. Their cringe-making fusspot behaviour is accepted as the norm in the USA, but when they do it here, waiters look very aggrieved - and so do we. However, in a way our American friends are right to ask for something different if that's what they want. A decent restaurant has plenty of alternatives in the kitchen and they can provide this. Sure, someone will have to adjust the bill and perhaps even charge us a bit more, but so what? Quality restaurants have a long menu, so pick the parts that you want and avoid the others. For instance, if they have knickerbocker glory on the menu, we can ask for the fruit, but not the cream and ice cream if that's how you want it.

You're in the money and you decide to go for a slap-up meal at a Harvester, Wheatsheaf or a similar type of restaurant. One unexpected danger is the soup, because the chef may well toss sugar into it to make it taste nice, so avoid thick soups, especially tomato soup (incidentally, a portion of canned tomato soup has over five spoons of sugar in it!) Unless you have a cholesterol problem, you can eat any main course, though if your cholesterol is high, choose poultry or fish rather than steak for your main course.

You can almost always order a side salad. This can be a small one for you alone or a large a Greek salad to share. If you're dieting, tell them not to put any dressing on, but to give you the cruet so that you can add the oil and vinegar yourself.

If you only eat out once a year, a bit of apple pie and custard or ice cream will probably be all right, but you must avoid obviously sugary things such as treacle tart, puddings with syrup and very chocolaty things like profiteroles. If your friends or partner have a dessert, take a spoonful of theirs!

Many people find that two courses are enough, so a starter and main meal may do the trick for you. If rolls and bread are on offer, choose brown or granary rather than white.

## *A Really Posh Restaurant*

You're rich or perhaps your ship has come in and you can afford to visit a very good restaurant. Avoid sole meunière (it's fried in butter) and opt for any low calorie, low cholesterol and low sugar option from the extensive menu. Avoid sauces and salad dressings if possible. Keep away from pâté, which is goose or pork liver with lots of fat. Don't eat rostis, because these are potatoes cooked in lots of goose fat.

It's always a good idea to sound out your waiter. You're condition is not unique, and the restaurant will probably be able to fit in with your requirements.

Choose a brown roll, granary or brown bread rather than white breads. Choose a starter and main course and skip the dessert, or ask for strawberries on their own.

## *A Carvery*

This is a buffet meat meal and it's a great option for a diabetic, although it isn't a great option for a vegetarian. Eat a big main course and don't bother with the dessert.

## *Going for an Indian*

There are more Indian restaurants in the UK than any other kind of eatery and many of us love Indian food. Most Indian food is fried in a lot of ghee (butter) or oil, but it's low GI, which is helpful. Select boiled rice rather than fried rice, along with chicken or lamb tikka or kebabs, because these dishes are not cooked in sauce and they aren't sweetened.

The other option is to eat whatever you like apart from dessert, but only "go for an Indian" very occasionally - say about once every couple of months. The same goes for takeaways, so you either keep to the boiled rice and tikka / kebab option, or eat Indian foods very rarely. All the trimmings are fattening, such as Peshawar naan, popadoms and chapattis. Such lovely food! Such a shame. But do have an Indian meal as a special treat once in a while.

### Chinese Nosh

Chinese food is a slightly better option than Indian food, because not all of it is sweet. Boiled rice goes well with Chinese food, so select that and avoid unnecessary calories. Avoid sweet and sour dishes and plum sauce. For instance, something like meat, chicken or prawns with bean sprouts, mushrooms, onions or cashew nuts should be fine. Even the addition of pineapple isn't too much of a problem. If the sweet and sour sauce comes in a pot rather than on the food, give the sauces to someone else and eat the pork, chicken or fritters in the batter with no sauce on them. The fact that they are fried makes them fattening, but at least you won't be adding sugar.

### Water

Drink plenty of water with the meal. If you have high blood pressure, drink still water rather than sparkling water, as that tends to have salts as well as minerals in it.

### A Doner Dinner

Doner lamb in pita bread is low in sugar but very high in fat - indeed, one kebab contains a whole day's fat requirement! Only eat this if there's absolutely nothing else available.

## Fish and Chips

A good trick is to get a larger portion of fish than you might ordinarily choose, and remove the batter. If you really do want to eat the batter, then restrict this meal to no more than once a month. The good news is that chip shop chips are normally made from potatoes rather than artificial ingredients.

## A Classic Burger Meal

A burger, chips and coke is a great choice to grab when you're out and about in the shopping centre and it doesn't cost the earth, either. Choose diet coke and a small burger rather than a "super-duper, double-decker, whopper, stomach stopper". Ask them to hold off any sauces. Avoid chicken nuggets, as they are fried in batter, and either do without the chips, or eat the chips and dump the bun.

## Kentucky Fried Chicken

Fried chicken is obviously fattening, and the addition of chips and coleslaw adds more calories. The chips are very salty. Only have such meals on very rare occasions.

## Filled Potatoes

This typifies some of the confusion of dealing with diabetes. Large, old potatoes are as high GI as white bread or sugar, but they do contain fibre and they aren't fried. You can lower the GI by filling them, but that's when you meet the next problem. The best filling is baked beans, although this is putting carbohydrate onto carbohydrate, but beans are also a form of protein. Other toppings are fatty (butter, cheese, mayo). Nevertheless, a filled spud is often a good option.

## Pub Grub

Although some things are not ideal, pub grub isn't too bad. If you have frequent pub lunches, eat your way around the menu, as that way you will have something of everything during the course of the month. The worst option is a ploughman's lunch, because it consists of a large lump of white bread, with fattening, salty cheese and sugared pickle.

## Sarnies

Sandwiches, rolls, baguettes and so on are fine, but choose granary or brown rolls or bread if possible. If there is nothing other than white bread on offer, go for chicken, ham or beef as a filling as that will slow the GI down. Marmite is good, as long as you like it and as long as you don't suffer from candida or thrush, because it is made from yeast, which is no good for those conditions.

## A Good Italian Restaurant

Italian food comes in various categories. One category that has all but disappeared is what I call a "proper restaurant" that would serve something like minestrone, antipasto or pasta to start with, followed by veal or liver with vegetables, after which, a laden dessert trolley would be wheeled to your table. While fattening, most of the starters and mains are fine, but the only "safe" dessert is fruit. However, if you only eat out once in a while and if your blood glucose isn't stratospheric, have some ice cream as a treat.

## Pizza and Pasta

Pizza bases contain white flour and sugar, so go for the thin and crispy rather than a deep pan pizza. Avoid those tempting balls of pizza bread. Choose a small dollop of tomato (and meat) sauce rather than a creamy carbonara sauce with your pasta.

## Thank God it's Friday!

This kind of American restaurant has loads of choice on the menu, so opt for lower calorie items, ask the waiter to hold the salad dressing, and choose a suitable dessert.

## Tapas

A tapas meal shouldn't be a problem, and if you can manage a San Miguel or two with it, so much the better - for the sheer pleasure of it.

## The Local Caff

Once in a while, Jan and I like to go to our local shopping parade, buy a couple of newspapers to read and then visit the café for bacon, egg and chips. A dietician would probably pass out on the floor in a dead faint at the very suggestion of this kind of meal, and there's nothing that we can say to recommend it, but we love our occasional café fry-up. It's inexpensive, enjoyable and sugar free.

## Meals on Wheels

The Social Services will provide meals on wheels suitable for diabetics, and they will even provide Halal, Kosher or other ethnic foods that are also diabetic-friendly.

## Cooked Supermarket Food

Jan and I often buy a cooked chicken from our supermarket, but in order to make sure the chicken doesn't have dextrose on it, we choose the barbeque chicken, which, in our area, is the only style that doesn't have dextrose added to it. Cooked ham hock is fatty, but all right on occasion.

## Drinks

We've covered the drink question elsewhere in this book, but let's go over some of it again here for restaurant purposes. Unfortunately, your only soft drink choices will probably be water, tomato juice or a diet cola. If you're an insulin dependent diabetic or if you're on heavy-duty pills, you must read the higher level books on diabetes and take specialist advice about alcohol, because alcoholic drinks can pose a problem with regard to hypoglycaemia. If you aren't sure what you should do, don't drink any alcohol.

### *Tea and Coffee*

If you use sweeteners in your tea and coffee, make sure you always have some in your bag or pocket. If you discover that you have forgotten your sweetener, ask if the café or restaurant has some available that you can use, because these days, many places do.

# 23

# Carbohydrates and Starches

*Carbohydrates ~ Useful Carbohydrates ~ Breads ~ Sugars ~ Sweeteners*

> *I went into McDonald's yesterday and said, "I'd like some fries".*
> *The girl at the counter said, "Would you like some fries with that?"*
> Jay Leno

To my mind, carbohydrates fall into two main categories, the first being filling foods and the second being sugary foods. "Fillers" are the things that usually form part of a meal and they are usually savoury. Some great carbs become a useful dessert item when you add sweeteners, such as rice pudding.

Some dieticians suggest that carbs should make up 50 to 60 per cent of our intake because they fill us up, but diabetics themselves say that this policy puts their blood glucose up too much and that they do much better by limiting their carbohydrate intake. Therefore, I suggest that you use carbs as part of your daily diet, but intersperse them with lots of leafy vegetables, salad and fruit, along with other foodstuffs.

### Useful Carbohydrates
~ New potatoes are lower GI than old ones.
~ Sweet potatoes, yams are lower GI and good for the brain.

~ Basmati rice is lower GI than the other kinds, but some people find it dry and hard to digest.

~ Easy-cook, long grain rice has now been found to be low GI.

~ Brown rice reminds me of hamster droppings, but it's low GI.

~ Couscous is made from a root and is all right as a change.

~ Cracked or bulgur wheat are nice as a "deli" salad ingredient.

~ Pasta is okay; brown or multicoloured pasta is even better.

~ Noodles are the same as pasta.

~ Canned sweet corn - look for tins that have no added sugar.

~ Corn on the cob.

~ Barley and rye that you can add to soup are good.

~ Sago, tapioca, semolina are fine.

~ Porridge.

~ Some breakfast cereals.

~ Popcorn - the kind you pop yourself with a little oil and very little salt added.

Carbs are often hidden in foods, like the padding in sausages, the coating on fish fingers and chicken Kiev, the breadcrumbs and flour in stuffing, and the thickeners in microwave foods and soups. Many snacks contain flour, such as sausage rolls, pork pies, cooked pies, pasties and steak and kidney pudding.

There are other foods that edge into the carb category, such as beans, swedes, parsnips, pumpkins and squashes as they also contain some carbohydrate. Some carbs have a high GI (swedes, parsnips and old potatoes) but these foods contain useful fibre, vitamins and minerals. Some fruit contains carbohydrates. Tropical fruits and melons have a higher GI than such things as apples and pears, but they contain loads of good vitamins and minerals, so they should form part of a varied diet.

Apparently, the GI climbs if food is over-cooked, so cook your pasta "al dente" and your potatoes and rice until done, but not overdone.

**NB:** The Glycaemic Index (GI) is based on white bread, which counts as 100 on the GI scale. Everything else is measured against this, so if something rates 50 on the GI scale, it takes twice as long for the sugar in it to be absorbed by the body, compared to white bread.

## Breads

The best choices are those that have a low GI and no added sugar, along with those that aren't eaten in bulk and that usually contain a filling, such as pita bread and wraps. The worst choice is a ploughman's lunch, as this includes a large lump of white bread that may contain added sugar.

### Good choices:

~ Granary bread
~ Wholemeal bread and rolls
~ Oat bread
~ Fancy breads with seeds in them, such as Burgins and Vogel
~ Wholemeal pita
~ White pita
~ Wraps
~ Brown bagels
~ Rye bread, with or without caraway seeds in it
~ Polish or Russian black bread
~ German pumpernickel breads
~ Ryvita crispbreads

### Poor choices

~ White bread
~ Fruit loaves
~ Brioches
~ That wonderful, plaited Jewish loaf called cholla
~ White bagels
~ Croissants contain white flour, fat and sugar
~ White breadsticks
~ Pretzels contain white flour and lots of salt, but they are a good occasional snack

## *Sugars*

These are the real baddies for a diabetic, so avoid them as much as possible.

~ Sugar of any colour or type
~ Icing sugar
~ Treacle
~ Syrup
~ Maple syrup
~ Honey
~ Glucose
~ Glucose syrup
~ Corn syrup
~ Molasses
~ Sorghum
~ Turbinado
~ Starch syrup
~ Malt extract
~ Dextrose
~ Maltodextrose
~ Sucrose

## *Sweeteners*

Sorbitol, maltitol and anything else ending with "ol" will give us diarrhoea if we eat more than a little of it. Fructose is low GI, so it is useful in cooking, while sucralose is now used as a non-fattening sweetener, as in Splenda. Some dieticians don't think much of fructose or the chemicals in sweeteners, but my feeling is that one has to tread a middle road and not become absolutely neurotic about our situation and ourselves.

*Now Here's a Treat*

The popcorn in packets that you put in the microwave usually has either a lot of salt in it or a lot of treacle, so buy the dried stuff and make it yourself. For the savoury variety, just put in very little salt. You can make a sweet variety by pouring a little agave nectar on the popped corn.

# 24

# Pulses

*Squeaky Beans ~ an easy Soup Recipe with Beans ~ Some other Ideas ~ Tips*

> *Beans, beans, good for the heart,*
> *The more you eat, the more you fart*

Children's playground song

Pulses are peas and beans. These can be fresh, dried, canned or frozen. There are over 50 different kinds of beans, and several different varieties of peas and lentils (lentils are dried peas). All are said to be good for the heart, and they are very good for diabetics as well.

Pulses are a weird food, because they are both carbohydrate (starch) and protein, although they contain less protein than meat. They are good fillers and they make a nice change. There are beans in all kinds of things, and they appear in canned or packet soups, such as pea soup or lentil soup.

The only danger that I know of, comes in the shape of dried red kidney beans, as these are toxic unless thoroughly cooked. Canned kidney beans are fine, as they have been thoroughly cooked.

If you're busy, here is a quick recipe that's good for the whole family:

~ Some baking potatoes
~ A can of mince
~ A small can of red kidney beans
~ Less than a quarter of a level teaspoon of chilli powder - use the mild variety if you're nervous
~ A packet of grated cheese - your favourite variety

*Method*
Bake the potatoes in the microwave for 8 to 10 minutes. If they are large, they might need more time than this, so use a fine knife to check that they are cooked through.

Put the mince in a saucepan and heat it through thoroughly, giving it a stir from time to time. Drain the can of beans, then toss them into the saucepan and stir in the chilli powder. Don't boil the mixture to death, but do cook it through thoroughly.

Open the packet of grated cheese and tip it into a dish to serve separately. Take the potatoes out of the microwave, put one on each plate and split each widely open, then pour the hot chilli onto the potatoes.

## Squeaky Beans
Runner beans, green beans and other fresh beans contain both the vegetable and the bean itself, so they are really good. The only problem here is that those little round green beans from Kenya tend to squeak when you chew them. My husband hates the squeaky effect so much that he won't eat them. I have no problem - I just ignore the squeaks!

## An Easy Soup Recipe with Beans
Take a can of chicken soup (the clear liquid broth type) or make up powdered chicken or vegetable stock that comes in a can, or make up a couple of Knorr cubes. There will be instructions somewhere on the packet. Soak dried butter beans, dried peas

or lentils for a few hours. Drain them in a sieve, run fresh water over them and cook them thoroughly until they are soft. Add the beans or lentils to the soup and heat it through. A quicker alternative is to drain a small can of butter beans and toss that in. Taste the soup before serving. Stock powders and cubes are salty, so you probably don't want to add more salt. This soup will fill you up without hurting the GI factor, and it's good value if you're on a budget. If you buy canned chicken soup with noodles, that's fine, too. Heat up a large can of chicken broth or chicken noodle soup. Open a very small can of garden peas, drain them and add them to the soup. If you add brown rolls with butter or spread, you and your family will enjoy an excellent snack lunch.

### Some Other Ideas

Use any type of canned beans or pre-soaked and rinsed dried beans to add to a casserole or stew. You can now tell your family that you're no longer serving stew, but cassoulet, which is much more impressive. I think there's a special type of bean that the French and Belgians put into cassoulet, but your husband and kids won't know any different (unless you have the misfortune to be married to a chef).

### Tips

If you buy canned beans and peas, choose those with no sugar and with reduced salt.

If you find beans "windy", only eat them when you aren't going to be out and about among other people. Drinking Actimel or Yoplait later in the day might help.

# 25

# Proteins

*Sources ~ Fish ~ Vegetable Proteins ~ Cheese ~ Milk ~ Cream ~ Butter ~ Trans Fat*

> *If more of us valued food and cheer and song*
> *above hoarded gold, it would be a merrier world.*

J. R. R. Tolkien.

## Sources

Protein usually comes from meat, poultry and fish, although there are some vegetable proteins. Most meat is fine, but processed foods, such as sausages, pork pies, delicatessen meats, salami and so on might contain things that are not great for you, such as starches, fats and salt. However, meat bothers some people, and if you are that way inclined, then don't eat meat.

To quote from nutritionist Sonia Jones in her book, "End the Food Confusion":

"Factory-farmed animals are fed food laced with antibiotics, chemicals, hormones, sawdust, paper pulp, and sometimes the remains of diseased animals. Chicks are so stuffed with chemicals that they grow so fast that their immature legs don't develop fast enough to hold this huge weight gain. What are all these additives doing to us or to our children?"

~ It may be better to buy meat from a farm, or at least to stick to organic meats if you can afford to do so.
~ Ensure that poultry is thoroughly cooked.
~ Only buy sausages that contain at least 70% meat.
~ Only eat deli food on occasion, since much of it is fatty.

## Fish

When you buy fish, ensure that the gills are red, the eyes clear and the flesh firm. Once you have bought it, cook it and eat it the same day. If the fish appears old or smells bad, don't buy it.

If you buy frozen meat, fish or poultry, thaw it out thoroughly, cook it as soon as practical and eat it immediately.

If you eat fish for lunch, you'll be alert during the afternoon, whereas lunchtime carbohydrates will make you sleepy.

Oily fish, such as salmon, mackerel, sardines and anchovies contain omega oils, which are good for your heart, organs and brain. Canned fish, by the way, is as good for you as fresh.

## Dairy - Cheese

Cheese contains protein, calcium, fat, carbohydrate and salt. It is good in moderation, but perhaps choose lower fat versions or cottage cheese some of the time.

## Dairy - Milk

My research shows that medical folk are in two minds about milk, with some saying that it is good, and others saying that it should be limited or even avoided. Milk contains fat, although the semi-skimmed and skimmed varieties are lower in fat than the full-cream type. Milk also contains carbohydrate sugars and lactic acid. I suggest that if you like milk, you should use it in tea, coffee, and desserts, or as an occasional drink in its own right. If you toss some cocoa powder and Splenda into a glass of milk, it becomes chocolate milk...lovely!

### Dairy - Cream

As you can imagine, cream is far too high in fat and cholesterol for good health, but nobody eats cream on a regular basis. Walls make a low sugar and low calory icecream, while Asda sell a diabetic icecream. Tesco sell a sugar-free custard powder. As usual, things may change, so always double check things for yourself.

### Dairy - Butter

Some nutritionists are violently against butter due to its fat and cholesterol content, while others say it is better for us than manufactured spreads. Perhaps buy a tub or packet of butter once in a while as a change from spreads, but spread it sparingly on bread or crisp-bread and don't cook with it, as you will then eat too much of it in one go.

### Hydrogenated Oils - Trans Fats

After doing some research, I discovered that some manufactured foods contain "trans fats". I discovered that these are made by forcing unpleasant chemicals into vegetable oil to make it thick and sticky. I read that some kinds of peanut butter contain this stuff and that one should check the jar in one's cupboard and toss it out if it lists hydrogenated oil in its ingredients. I looked in my cupboard, discovered that my peanut butter did indeed contain this material, so I binned it.

There is currently no legal requirement for labelling foods with trans-fat or hydrogenation information, but this will very likely change, because these "bad" fats raise your "bad" cholesterol level.

A website called www.moodfoodcompany.co.uk sells nut spreads without trans-fats, among many other interesting products.

Some gluten-free health products contain trans fats.

# 26

# Fruit and Vegetables

---

*Sasha's Tips ~ Dried Fruit ~ Canned and Frozen Fruit and Veggies ~ Bowel Cancer ~ Dig for Victory*

*The only way to keep your heath is to eat what you don't want, drink what you don't like and do what you'd rather not.*
Mark Twain

All fruit, salads and vegetables are good. Some of these are quite sweet and they may register fairly high on the GI scale, but the modern view is that they are fine, because they also provide vegetable fibre, which has been shown to be a beneficial food constituent for diabetics. The higher GI foods are parsnips, swedes, melons, grapes and bananas, but as long as you eat a variety of veggies, salads and fruits, you aren't likely to overdose on any one of them. A mixed bag of foods give you a wide variety of natural sugars, vitamins, trace elements, anti-toxicants and other goodies.

The buzzword is to eat foods of different colours, and to eat five items of fresh foods a day. These can be a mix of fruit, salad or vegetables. A smoothie or fruit drink counts as one item, but make your own, because commercial smoothies tend to have high sugar and calorie levels.

### Sasha's Tips
~ Give schoolchildren a piece of fruit or some cherries in their lunch bag on most days.
~ Take a piece of fruit to work with you.
~ If you have bad teeth or dentures, you may find it hard to bite into apples or pears, so cut them up and nibble pieces.

### Dried Fruit
Although dried fruit is better than sweets and chocolates it can be very high in sugar, so only have a little at a time. The worst offenders are dates and figs, because not only do they contain sugar, but they are often also preserved in treacle. Look for fresh figs and dates that come from Israel, these are better for you.

### Canned and Frozen Fruit and Veggies
These are all good to eat and they count towards our five items a day. Ensure that your canned peas, beans and sweetcorn don't contain added salt or sugar. Check that the sugar content is below 6g per 100g.

Choose fruit in juice, but drain the juice off before using the fruit. Tins of apple and other fruits that are intended for pies may be packed with sugar.

### Bowel Cancer
Moving on from diabetes for a moment, to the greatest scourge in this country at present, I have to mention cancer, and especially bowel cancer. When a person eats badly, the bowel doesn't clear properly and polyps can develop. These polyps eventually end up as bowel cancer. By eating roughage in the form of vegetables, fruit, wholegrain bread, wholegrain pasta, porridge and drinking lots of water, you can help to keep this disease at bay.

### Dig for Victory
Short and sweet - growing your own salad and veg is fun!

# 27

# Drinks

---

*Alcohol ~ Department of Health Information ~ Good Drinks ~ Wine ~ Beer ~ What to Avoid ~ The Good News ~ Mixers ~ Hypoglycaemia ~ Some Cocktail Ideas ~ Soft Drinks ~ Hot Drinks*

> *A man's got to believe in something;*
> *I believe I'll have another drink.*

W. C. Fields

### Alcohol

Fortunately, you can drink alcohol with diabetes, but you should stick to the health guidelines, which are a maximum of 14 units a week for women and 21 units a week for men. Young people and the elderly should drink less. You should have some alcohol-free days each week, and you shouldn't drink your whole allowance in one go.

The information in this chapter comes from the Department of Health and other "official-type" sources, along with some from diabetics themselves.

*The Department of Health Information*

| DRINK | UNITS |
|---|---|
| One pint, ordinary lager | 2 |
| One pint, strong lager | 3 |
| One pint, ordinary bitter | 2 |
| One pint, best bitter | 3 |
| One pint, ordinary cider | 2 |
| One pint, strong cider | 3 |
| 125ml red or white wine 12% alcohol | 1.5 |
| 175ml red or white wine 14% alcohol | 2.5 |
| Pub measure, spirits (25ml) | 1 |
| Large pub measure, spirits (35ml) | 1.5 |
| Double measure spirits | 2 |
| Alcopop | 1.5 |

## Good Drinks

Spirits are better than wine and beer as they can be stretched with mixers, but you must remember to ask for sugar-free mixers. Dry sherry is fine and several diabetics have told me that they do well on vodka, gin or whisky.

## Wine

Years ago, the diabetes clinic in St Mary's hospital in Paddington used to tell their patients that white wine is better than red wine as they said that it contains less sugar. Since then, scientists have discovered that the colour makes no difference, but what does make a difference is the sweetness of the wine.

~ If you want to make a long drink, you can make up a spritzer with white wine and soda water, or Dry Martini and sugar-free lemonade

~ Apparently Australian Shiraz Sangovese Rosé is low in alcohol and calories

~ Weight Watchers market a low calorie sparkling wine

## Beer

Diabetics tell me that Pilsner is the best beer for them as it has less sugar. Carlsberg is also supposed to be low calorie, and therefore a better choice of lager. I drink beer and lager so rarely that I don't worry about the type I am drinking.

## What to Avoid

~ Alcopops. These are specially made to appeal to youngsters, so they are basically sugar-pop drinks with alcohol added

~ Cocktails

~ Liqueurs

~ Port

~ Medium or sweet sherry

~ Late harvest or other sweet wine, such as Sauternes

~ Special drinks such as Galliano or Lemoncello

### The Good News

I found some Bacardi Breezers in the supermarket the other day, labelled "half sugar". The sugar content is well below the 6g per 100g level, so I bought a pack of four as an experiment. I chose the pomegranate variety, and it is very nice.

### Mixers

It's easy to buy a variety of sugar free or "light" soft drinks that you can use as mixers for the home, but it not easy to find them when you're out. The following are the only ones that I've seen in pubs:

~ Water
~ Mineral water
~ Soda water
~ Diet Cola
~ Slimline tonic
~ Tomato juice

If your pub isn't a large or busy one and if your publican is helpful, you could ask him/her to make you up a highball, which is a glass of ice with whisky or vodka poured over it. In the case of the vodka, you might like to add a slice of lemon or lime. If you're a regular, it might be worth asking the publican to keep some diet mixers for you, such as sugar-free lemonade and sugar-free bitter lemon. Alternatively, you might buy them yourself and ask if the publican would keep a couple of cans in his cooler for you. A lovely drink is a sugar free ginger beer called "_Light_ Fiery Jamaican Ginger Beer". With that, you can ask the barman to make you a Whisky Mac. Lovely…

> **The only place I've seen that sells "Light, Fiery, Jamaican Ginger Beer" is Waitrose.**

*Hypoglycaemia*

Alcohol poses specific problems for diabetics, because it doesn't mix well with the pills or insulin injections as these lower the blood glucose level in the body. Alcohol lowers it even more, so it's possible for a diabetic to become extremely ill with a "hypo". Once the blood glucose level starts to sink, it can keep on sinking for up to 16 hours, which is why some diabetics die in their sleep. You need more advice than I'm giving you here, so look at the bibliography at the back of this book for more in-depth books on diabetes, and consult your dietician and diabetes nurse.

| DRINK | CALORIES |
|---|---|
| Pint, Bitter, canned and draught | 91 |
| Pint, Bitter, keg | 88 |
| Pint, Mild bitter, draught | 71 |
| Pint, Brown ale | 80 |
| Pint, Pale ale | 91 |
| Bottled stout | 105 |
| Pint, strong ale (barley wines) | 205 |
| Pint, Lager - ordinary strength | 85 |
| Pint, sweet cider | 110 |
| Pint, dry cider | 95 |
| Glass, red wine | 85 |
| Glass, rosé wine, medium | 89 |
| Glass, sweet white wine | 118 |
| Glass, dry white wine | 83 |
| Glass, medium white wine | 94 |
| Glass, sparkling white wine | 95 |
| Small glass, port | 79 |
| Small glass, dry sherry | 58 |

### Some Cocktail Ideas

~ Vodka, diet cola and a slice of lemon or lime
~ Gin and Slimline tonic or sugar free orange
~ Lime juice and soda water
~ Vodka and sugar free orange. (This cocktail is called a Screwdriver)
~ Malibu, a little pineapple juice and sparkling water
~ Diet pomegranate and Bacardi
~ Bacardi and diet cola. (This one's called a Cuba Libra)
~ Black coffee and vodka
~ Grenadine and orange or lemon

### Soft Drinks

We in Britain are lucky, because we're blessed with an astonishing choice of sugar free and no-added-sugar drinks. This may also be the case in the USA, but it's not so in Europe. I suggest that you roam around several supermarket soft drink departments, because each supermarket stocks something different.

You can drink these things alone or make a cocktail out of them, with or without alcohol, such as a St. Clements, which consists of orange and lemon juice. Make up tall glasses of diluted, no-added-sugar squashes with ice, a slice of orange and a slice of lemon and perhaps a sprig of mint. Add a swizzle stick and you will have a great alcohol-free cocktail that even children can enjoy.

Diabetics, dieters and those who have other health issues are all told to drink lots of water every day, and I've heard amounts ranging from two litres a day to 12 glasses a day! Blimey, that sounds like the Chinese water torture! Sure, if you have a severe kidney complaint or if you're fighting off an attack of cystitis, it's essential to drink a lot of water for a while. In normal circumstances, I suggest that you take a 1.5 litre bottle of water with you to work and sip or drink it throughout the day until it's gone.

Pure fruit juice is usually very high in sugar, but you can always dilute it.

## *Hot Drinks*

For many years, Americans have made a great fuss about coffee being harmful. I've even seen films (presumably based on real life) where the parents had hysterics upon discovering that their school-age child had made himself a cup of coffee. I guess that drinking dozens of cups of American-style coffee a day is harmful due to the caffeine content, let alone the cream. Latte coffee is very milky, very sweet and very comforting, which is why it's so popular, but it's extremely high in calories and too sugary for a diabetic. Oddly enough, espresso and other very strong types of coffee contain less caffeine than standard types. Decaffeinated coffee is said to have chemicals in it, due to the caffeine extraction method. All in all, coffee seems to be a bad choice, but I believe in the middle way, so I suggest that you drink any type of coffee that you like, but no more than two cups a day.

Tea is a good choice, especially if you drink it black or Russian style, with a slice of lemon. It rehydrates and lowers blood glucose.

It's okay to make hot chocolate, but you will have to buy black cocoa and use lots of sweeteners with plenty of hot milk to make it palatable. Other hot drinks might be Ribena, water with lemon juice and sweeteners, and Bovril or soup in a cup. Check the labels for soups as some contain sugar, and cuppa soups have a lot of starchy thickener in them, so only have one of these every other day. Some products are salty, so take care if you have high blood pressure.

A large variety of herbal drinks are available, including chamomile, raspberry leaf, forest fruits and so on; these shouldn't do you any harm, so if you like these drinks, they make a nice change. It is really a matter of taste. Something that's popular in South Africa and is making its way over here is "rooibos tea", which translates from Afrikaans as "redbush tea".

It doesn't dehydrate and it doesn't contain caffeine or tannin, so it's said to be very good for you. Personally I can't stand it. I can't bear chamomile tea, either. Oddly enough, I do like Chinese green tea, because I have spent quite a lot of time in China and I learned to enjoy it there. "Chac'un à son goût", as they say.

# 28

# Body Care

---

*Eyes ~ Skin ~ Hands ~ Heart ~ Bladder ~ Constipation ~ Diarrhoea ~ Bad Breath ~ Look After Your Tootsies ~ Hair ~ Over the Counter Medicines*

> *The feet are the gateway to 10,000 illnesses.*

Japanese proverb

This is intended to be a very simple book that focuses on day-to-day care, so I suggest that you buy one or two of the more "medical" books if you want to know full details about the nasties that can happen to a diabetic. If anything bothers you or gets out of hand, please consult your doctor or your diabetic nurse, but there are simple steps that you can take to avoid problems, or sort out mild ones.

### *Eyes*
Diabetes affects the eyes in various ways. In the short term, vision can become blurred, because the fluid in the eyeball responds to changes in glucose levels, and if your glucose count is fluctuating, your eyes will find it hard to keep up.

If your eyes get dry, ask your doctor for advice. He may well recommend Visco Tears as a lubricant. Cigarette smoking is a problem, as the smoke gets into the eyes and dries them.

Smoking aggravates conjunctivitis and sties, and the sugar in the body encourages bacteria to flourish along the eyelids.

A bigger problem is diabetic retinopathy, which leads to blindness. Read the books that I've listed in the bibliography to learn more about this problem.

As a diabetic in the UK, you can have a free eye test once a year. If you're not on medication (i.e. not registered as a diabetic) and you're under sixty, you will pay for the test, but it's not expensive and it could save your eyesight.

You may or may not be able to use contact lenses, so discuss this with your optician.

## Skin

The skin is the largest organ in your body and it responds badly to many ailments. Diabetes can make cuts and zits hard to heal. Use liquid hand and face wash or whatever simple soap your skin can tolerate. Have a facial (yes, they do men too), and ask the beautician about products that will help your skin to stay in good condition. The sugar in your sweat can set up infections, so shower or bathe every day.

Most aggravating are the soreness and sensitivity that come when even a little superfluous glucose is swimming around in your system. I find that seams under the arms of shirts and tee-shirts sometimes make me sore. Cheaper garments are often made with plastic stitching or strips of plastic in the seams, and these become sharper once the garment has been washed. Bras can become so uncomfortable that you spend a fortune hunting for one that doesn't feel like an instrument of torture. Buy more tee-shirts and underwear than you need, so that you can throw stuff out when it starts to cause trouble.

Many diabetics suffer from dry skin, so you might want to use face cream and body lotion at times. Oddly enough, this has a beneficial spin-off effect. I once remember reading a magazine article about skin care, in which the journalist said that she had researched the subject by going to old people's homes. While in the homes, she asked the women whose skin looked the best what they had done over the years. Every one of them said they had always used the simplest soap or cleanser, and they had always used moisturiser after washing their faces.

I read in one American book that diabetics shouldn't use saunas. The author didn't say why this was, so if you happen to be a billionaire diabetic and you are considering fitting a sauna into your house, it might be worth looking into this before calling in the builders.

### Hands

Cuts and scrapes can take a long time to heal and they can become infected. If you cut or scrape yourself, put on Savlon, Germolene or something similar.

If you burn yourself, plunge the hand into cold water for ten minutes, then wrap it in a clean towel and go to a nurse, your doctor or even to hospital.

Diabetic hands get cold and this makes the skin dry, making the hands even more susceptible to cuts and broken skin. Use loads of hand cream, as this gives a measure of protection. Ask your friends to give you hand and face cream for birthdays, Christmas or some other occasion.

Another great present that people can buy is a pair of fleecy gloves. Keep gloves in the pockets of every coat and jacket you own, so that if the weather changes, you're prepared. Now here's a really radical idea - keep a pair of gloves in the glove compartment of your car!

Use rubber gloves, gardening gloves and protective gloves when working on the car or doing DIY.

### Heart

Do everything you can to lower your cholesterol level. Keep your blood pressure down by avoiding unnecessary salt. Take enough regular exercise.

### *Bladder*

Attacks of cystitis can create sores and scars in the bladder. Here are some ideas:

~ If your bladder is "sensitive", Tena and Boots Own pads are useful.

~ Keep your diabetes under control.

~ Keep packets of cystitis powders in your home, also at your place of work and in your suitcase when you travel.

~ At the first sign of cystitis, start taking the medication.

~ If you don't have cystitis powders available, buy bicarbonate of soda and plonk a level teaspoonful in a glass of water. It doesn't taste good, but it will help.

~ Avoid drinking fruit juice and avoid eating citrus fruit and tomatoes for a while.

~ Wear cotton undies and avoid tights for a while.

### *Constipation*

A change in diet can cause constipation. Here are some tips:

~ Buy a packet of bran and sprinkle a little onto any kind of breakfast cereal.

~ Eat an apple a day and/or dried prunes for a few days, until your body sorts itself out.

~ Dehydration can cause constipation; that's a problem for many diabetics, so drink more water and other fluids, and cut out alcohol for a while.

Another good trick is to dance around the house, because this gets things moving. Do the cha cha while you're making dinner, or do some running on the spot while making the bed. Pinch the kids' skipping rope and skip in the garden. Do belly dancing or any other kind of dancing that makes you wiggle your hips. Men should pretend they're wriggling their booty in Kylie Minogue's dance troupe, a rap troupe or on Strictly Come Dancing, or doing a "Michael Jackson" moonwalk. Your family and neighbours will probably recommend a visit to a psychiatrist, but your bowels will start to move!

## *Diarrhoea*

You may get a loose bowel due to changing your diet. Eat eggs and mashed potatoes for a while and avoid foods that scratch or aggravate the bowel. If the diarrhoea doesn't clear up after a few days, go to the doctor.

## *Bad Breath*

This is a sign that your diabetes isn't doing well, so please get a check up. For mild cases, drink some water and chew some sugar-free gum. You can get sprays for fresh breath as well. Brush your teeth at least twice a day, and use Tee Pee brushes (ask at the chemist's) to brush between the teeth, to clear out mucky debris. Your mouth is susceptible to infection now, so you must keep it clean. An electric toothbrush with lots of nice clean heads is a good idea - and this can be yet another birthday or Christmas present idea for those who don't know what to buy you.

## *Look After Your Tootsies*

The things that can go wrong with a diabetic's feet aren't at all nice. Read the books listed in the bibliography to discover just how much trouble you can attract. The tingling, burning and stabbing pains that diabetics get in their feet at night, are due to damage to the nerve endings. After a while, the nerves die and the feet no longer feel pain. That's very dangerous, because a tiny stone (even a large grain of sand) in a shoe or a badly fitting shoe, can rub a hole or make a blister that bursts and gets infected. A wounded foot will take a very long time to heal - if it heals at all.

When I was a child, I caught the back of my heel on a piece of rusty metal. The wound turned septic, and whatever my mother or I tried, we couldn't get it to heal. The wound just got larger and messier, until the whole of my right heel was a suppurating mess. When I got to hospital, the nurse poured some magic powder on my poor heel and within a day, the wound started to heal properly. The powder was something that we had only heard of, but never seen, and it was called penicillin. The first real test of penicillin had been on wounded soldiers in the Second World War, and it had proved itself there. The magic powder certainly saved my foot, and maybe even my life.

The over-sensitivity is better, because it shows that things are still working, but it's caused by the deterioration of the nerves and small veins.

### *Here are some tips for basic every-day care:*

~ Never walk around barefoot, because you might damage yourself without noticing. Even if you can still feel pain and pressure on your feet, things don't heal quickly when you're diabetic. Wear slippers, sandals or something around the house.

~ Before putting on shoes, boots or wellies, tip them up and shake them out. Soldiers in the desert do this in case a scorpion has crawled into their boots at night. In your case, you don't need anything as nasty as a scorpion to cause you trouble, because even a piece of grit lurking in the shoe can be dangerous.

~ Go to an old-fashioned shoe shop and have your feet measured. Shops that specialise in good shoes for children will have measuring plates, and as long as you don't go on a busy Saturday or just before a new school year, the assistant should be happy to help. You might be surprised to find that your foot size has changed. Some people's feet spread as they get older; others go down a size when they lose weight.

~ Buy the best quality shoes you can afford. Buy trainers and decent flatties for general wear. Don't wear shoes when they are truly worn out. If you only spend real money on shoes and socks and buy everything else cheapo, you will be doing yourself a favour.

~ Make sure your shoes are long and wide enough, but not so loose that you slither around in them.

~ If you're a young and fashion conscious girl, keep your fancy shoes for dates, outings, clubbing, pubbing and so on. Wear trainers or other covered-up shoes when you don't need to look especially good. Never dance in open-toed shoes.

~ Wear trainers or flatties to get to work, and keep something nicer in your drawer or locker to change into. If you travel on public transport, this will really save your feet.

~ Think hard about sandals and flip-flops when on holiday. On the one hand, your feet will feel hot in covered up shoes, but on the other hand, your toes can be too vulnerable in sandals. This might be a case of wearing something like plimsolls while going to the beach and then changing into flip-flops when you're there.

~ Keep your feet in the shade as much as possible, and use plenty of sunscreen lotion on them.

~ If you find it hard to make a good job of cutting your toenails, go to a chiropodist.

~ Wash your feet every day and dry them carefully, especially between your toes.

~ Never put a pair of socks back on once you have taken them off, even if you have only had them on for a couple of hours. Put on a clean pair.

~ Modern socks often contain elastic matter that shrinks after several washes, then the heel doesn't fit properly and the toes become compressed. When this starts to happen, throw the socks away. Whatever your age, people are always happy to buy something simple like socks for your birthday, Christmas or some other occasion. Ask everyone to buy you socks. If your legs are fat, ask them to check that the socks won't be too tight around the ankle.

~ A good tip that my non-diabetic husband suggests is to turn socks inside out if they have the kind of seam that rubs on the tops your toes. He does this with such socks simply because he finds the seam uncomfortable, but if you can't feel the rubbing, it can soon turn your toes raw.

~ Inspect your feet every day. Use a mirror on the floor to check under your soles.

~ If you get even the slightest bit of athlete's foot, zap it right away with an over-the-counter product.

~ Use a moisturiser on the tops and soles of your feet, but don't put it between your toes.

~ Girls and women may use nail lacquer on their toenails, because this will make them focus on their feet.

~ If you have a verruca, visit a podiatrist or chiropodist - it may be best to leave it alone rather than treating it.

~ Don't sit around for long with your legs or feet crossed. Wriggle your feet and toes around from time to time to keep the circulation going.

## *Hair*

Use good quality shampoos and conditioners to combat dryness and prevent hair breaking off or falling out. Don't dye or perm your hair if it's falling out. Put in streaks so that you don't dye too close to the roots. If you can't stand going without hair colour, try to leave it for as long as possible between tints.

## *Over the Counter Medicines*

Choose sugar free throat tablets and cough medicines. Read the labels and the paperwork that comes with all medicines to ensure that it's right for you. Some vitamin supplements are not good for diabetics. Wart remover can be dangerous, especially if you use it on a verruca. Look, think and don't barge ahead without reading the instruction leaflet in the packet.

# 29

# Oh, God, It's Christmas!

*The Christian Calendar ~ Problem Food ~ If You Overdo
Things ~ A Clever Woman*

> *Health is the thing that makes you think that
> now is the best time of the year.*

Franklin Pierce Adams

## *The Christian Calendar*

The Christian calendar used to celebrate twelve days of
Christmas, and that idea now seems to have been resurrected,
although no longer for religious reasons. When I was young,
Christmas lasted two days - Christmas Day and Boxing Day -
and if either fell on a weekend, that was just hard luck, because
we didn't get any days off in lieu, but now the holiday seems to
go on forever. The main pressure falls onto women, and it starts
several weeks before the holiday itself. Stress is a killer for
diabetics, so do all you can to minimise it.

## *Problem Food*

Food is more of a problem for diabetics at Christmas than at
other times because so many Christmas treats are sweet.
Fortunately, not everything is bad for you. Starters, main
courses, salads and buffet foods or supper foods are usually fine,
and if you're the cook, you can make a dessert for yourself that

suits your needs, such as strawberries and cream. If someone else is cooking, ask them to fix you up with some fruit salad.

### Here are some other tips:

~ Make mince pies from scratch by buying dried fruit and making small pies.
~ Make vegetable crudités.
~ Buy some nuts - preferably not peanuts as they are so fattening.
~ Buy crisps made of real potatoes, and Weight Watchers' Hoops.
~ Ask friends and relatives not to push "bad" food on to you.
~ Avoid eating sweet things in the run-up to Christmas, so that you can allow yourself one piece of "real cake" or a small portion of Christmas pudding on the day.

### If You Overdo Things

~ If you eat the wrong thing, drink a few glasses of water and walk around the block a couple of times.
~ Don't drink alcohol on an empty stomach, and never binge. Check your blood glucose and take steps if the level starts dropping.
~ If you're in the habit of nibbling leftovers from the children's plates, squirt washing up liquid on them - that will stop you in your tracks.
~ Avoid cranberry sauce, because it contains a huge amount of sugar.
~ Focus on all the lovely things that you *can* eat, rather than getting bent out of shape about the things you can't eat.

### A Clever Woman

Since writing this, I have just chatted to Karen, who I know always has at least 25 people at her home for Christmas Day. Karen is not a diabetic, so she has ample energy, but she also has a full time business of her own, three teenage children and a not-very-well husband. So how does she do it? Does she wave a wand and shout - Harry Potter style - "Refectorium Mass de Cristos Festorius?" Well, almost.

Karen's mother is her housekeeper, and at Christmas, Karen's mother makes sure that the house is clean and the veggies are prepared. Karen's husband does all their Christmas shopping and cooking. Karen's children have been trained never to sit around and be waited on, so they put up the tree, decorate it and hang decorations around the house. Karen's friends and family bring contributions of food, drinks and snacks with them. Karen told me that she loves having her family around and that she always has a great time at Christmas. I'm not surprised!

Psychologists tell us that Christmas is the time when women traditionally prove how praiseworthy and admirable they are, by providing a perfect holiday for their families. If so, Karen scores nil points on the praiseworthy and admirable list, but 100 points on the clever woman list.

At the end of the day, you will have to forego some of the foods and treats that others eat, but remember that you're not alone, because there are people with cholesterol problems, stomach ulcers, alcohol problems and allergies who also have to forego things. There's an upside to this, because you will gain less weight over the holidays than your non-diabetic friends.

# 30

# Travel and Holidays

---

*Safety First ~ Come Fly With Me - Travel Tips ~ Feet and Holidays ~ Glucose and Heat ~ The Travails of the Travel Trail ~ Third World Countries ~ Goods From Overseas ~ Emigration ~ Food and Holidays*

> *In an undeveloped country, don't drink the water.*
> *In a developed one, don't breath the air.*

Jonathan Raban

A holiday should be fun. It should offer a change of pace and a change of scene, and you should come back refreshed and with happy memories. What you don't need is for your holiday to be ruined by a silly accident, which means taking some extra precautions.

## *Safety First*

Wear a MedicAlert or similar bracelet or pendant, and put any details about your ailment, prescription or anything else of the kind in your purse or wallet. If you would like some laminated cards saying whatever you think is necessary, you should be able to have them made up at your local print shop. If you can't do that for any reason, we may be able to help; email Jan on info@zampub.com and put the words "diabetes cards" in the subject line, so that we don't delete it as spam. We have to charge a little for this, and we can't guarantee we will always have a laminator on hand, but we like to help if we can.

Get a card that says "diabetic" in the local language. Here it is, in a few more common languages. Where I happen to know the feminine versions, I've given them.

| "DIABETIC" IN OTHER LANGUAGES | |
|---|---|
| French: | Diabétique |
| German: | Diabetetiker / Diabetetike |
| Italian: | Diabetico / Diabetica |
| Norwegian: | Sukkersyke |
| Polish: | Chory na cukrzyçe |
| Portuguese: | Diabetico/ Diabeticia |
| Serbo/Croat: | Dijabeticar |
| Spanish: | Diabetico/ Diabetica |
| Swedish: | Diabetiker |

## *Come Fly With Me - Travel Tips*

My daughter, Helen, worked for several airlines over many years and she assures me that all airlines will provide a diabetic meal (the airline code for this is DBML). Book the meal when you book the holiday or flight. If you can't be bothered to pre-order a special meal, eat everything except the dessert. The roll or sandwich will be white, but it's only small, so it probably won't hurt too much. Here are some other tips:

~ Drink water or tomato juice on the flight.
~ Avoid all alcohol before and while flying.
~ If you travel on a budget holiday airline, you have to buy sandwiches on the plane, so it makes good sense to prepare your own packed lunch instead. Remember that at present,

some airlines won't let you take much water or other liquids with you, so you will have to buy that in-flight.

~ If you are on insulin, get top-dollar travel insurance and state clearly that you have diabetes on the form. Check the small print / terms and conditions carefully, as some insurers specifically exclude certain conditions, such as diabetes, from the policy. Go elsewhere if you have to, but make sure that your diabetes is covered, even if the premium is higher.

~ Get letters from your doctor to take along, if you need to carry syringes with you on the flight. Make several photocopies of these letters and keep them in several places in your bags and luggage. Make copies of your prescription in case you need to get medicines while you're away. Some countries, such as Singapore, want to see medical evidence of your condition if you carry syringes and insulin with you.

~ Take double the amount of medicines that you think you will need, in case something gets broken or lost, or in case you need more than usual.

~ Never pack essential medication cases into the luggage compartment. This is partly in case your luggage goes missing and partly because the extreme temperatures will destroy insulin and it may affect other drugs too.

~ When you get to your hotel, put most of your "works" and pills in the safe and only carry around what you need for the day.

~ List all your necessary medicines, not just your diabetic ones, including bandages, ointments, etc. on a check sheet, and tick everything off as you pack. If you travel a lot, make up a permanent travel kit of medicines and keep the stuff in it up to date. Make several copies of a general travel checklist so that you don't have to rely on memory each time you go away.

~ If you cross time zones and need to inject or take medicines at certain intervals, try to keep this up as best you can.

~ Tell the cabin crew that you have syringes on you. You may have to give them to the stewardess and then get them back from her when needed.

~ If you intend to do something sporty or arduous, it would be best to go with a friend or in a group, especially if the environment is likely to be "challenging" (e.g. desert, jungle, mountains, arctic). Tell your companions about your condition.

~ If you go somewhere hot (or cold) for your holiday, pack a cool bag to keep your medicines and blood testing kit in.

~ If you get a tummy bug, drink still bottled water with lemon juice and a sweetener in it. Test your blood frequently.

### *Feet and Holidays*

Everybody's feet are vulnerable to accidents when on holiday, because we walk more than usual, and we do so over rougher ground than usual. Foreign streets are often not paved as well or as evenly as they are in the UK. In addition to the foot care advice that I've given earlier, here are some extra tips:

~ It's liberating to wear sandals and flip-flops, and it must be even more so for a man, because men so rarely go around without shoes or trainers. Girls and women love wearing mules, sandals and pretty flip-flops. I just love them all, but I know from bitter experience that if I walk about on rough ground, I need flatties or trainers. Without proper support, I will surely turn an ankle or bash my foot and end up with a cut.

~ If you want to harden your toes and feet before a holiday, dab them with surgical spirit on a bit of cotton wool every day for a month before the off.

~ Your feet will swell in hot climates and when going in and out of air-conditioning, so ensure that your holiday shoes or sandals are not too snug a fit.

~ Ensure that hiking boots well broken in before your trip, and take plenty of changes of socks and some moisturising cream for your feet in your backpack.

~ Never go anywhere without a couple of plasters and some ointment in your bag.

~ When travelling to and from your destination, wear comfortable, roomy old shoes, especially if you have to fly.

~ If you're in an area where you might walk on a sea urchin or some other underwater hazard, buy those very thick-soled plastic sandals and wear them while you're in the water or wandering around on the beach.

~ Take changes of shoes and sandals with you, even if it means having less weight allowance for other things.

~ Always shake out shoes before putting them on, in case there's a bit of grit in them. Your feet may not be sensitive enough to feel grit, so you could develop a nasty wound without being aware of it.

~ Be very cautious about buying shoes in holiday places and markets in countries like Spain and Italy. They are often really cheap, but many of them are poor quality and fit. At best, you will dump them in the bin before long and at worst, they can hurt or damage your feet. Where shoes are concerned, remember the old saying, "cheap is dear".

~ If you do buy good shoes and you want to wear them right away, keep an old pair of shoes in your bag to change into if the newies start to rub.

~ If you're in a sunny place, lather yourself and your feet all over with top-quality, factor-50 suntan cream. Think about it - your feet don't see daylight most of the time, and therefore the sun will burn them more swiftly than any other exposed part of your body when on holiday. Use waterproof sunscreen if you intend going into the sea or a swimming pool. When you come out of the water, shove another load of suntan lotion on, and don't forget to plonk plenty onto the soles of your feet and the undersides of your toes, because if

you doze off on the beach, even if under the shade of an umbrella, these exposed areas will pick up a lot of UV light.
~ Standing around in shallow seawater in the sun will magnify the sun's strength and give you sunburn and blisters on your feet. This will easily ruin your holiday, and it might even end up ruining your life. Make sure you put loads of high-quality suntan lotion on before you go into shallow water.
~ If you're going to be in a grassy area where there are likely to be stinging insects or even snakes or scorpions, wear full-cover shoes, never sandals; boots may even be a better idea.
~ Let's say that you're a girl or a woman, you've bought some really special shoes for a wedding or for some other special occasion, and you need to wear them in a bit, so that you don't end up with a rub or a blister. Pull a pair of old pop-socks over them to avoid scuffs, and then walk about in them at home.
~ A man should walk about in new sandals or shoes indoors several times before the holiday, to wear them in.
~ If you go clubbing and you want to wear heels or sandals, take a large bag along and stuff a pair of soft flatties in it, then you can change for the trip home and give your feet a break.
~ If you aren't happy about a foot wound, ask the hotel or ask around for a doctor.
~ If you're going on a ski-ing, skating, snowboarding holiday or anything else that requires special footwear, buy your own footwear before you go rather than hiring at the venue. Hiring shoes that someone else has worn will save money, but it might cost you your legs.

This doesn't really have anything to do with diabetes, but it's a good tip for reducing the weight of your case for your trip back home. Wear clothes and shoes that are at the end of their lives for the journey out or for days out where your appearance doesn't matter, then dump them in a bin somewhere and don't bring them back.

### *Glucose and Heat*

Hot weather and changes of temperature can interfere with your glucose levels, so you might need to test yourself more frequently and adjust the dose of your pills or your injections. Drink plenty of water and create a balance between being active and resting.

The stress of travel might affect your blood glucose, so you must take this into account as well. Ask your health specialist about what you can do when travelling across time zones.

If you're a diet-controlled diabetic, you still need to drink lots of water and sugar free drinks - even more so perhaps than those who can adjust drug doses.

Alcohol dehydrates you, and it can lower the glucose level too much for those on insulin or pills, so add plenty of mixers to your drinks or intersperse soft drinks with your alcoholic drinks.

It may not be easy to get sugar-free soft drinks in some places. If you're travelling by anything other than a plane, you can take some Robinson's no-added-sugar fruit drink to add to the local bottled water. Drink as much water and black tea or lemon tea as you can. You may be able to get diet cola in many places around the world, but if you're going from civilisation into a remote area, take some cans or small bottles of water with you.

Take some glucose sweets along at all times.

Diabetics who are seriously ill, especially type 1 diabetics, must be aware of the effects of heat and alcohol - and so must your companions. They must be aware of the signs of too much or too little glucose, and they must know what to do about it. If necessary, go to hospital.

For those with a lower degree of diabetes, if you drink alcohol on an empty stomach, eat some glucose or a sweet, drink some water, then order up a sandwich or eat a proper meal.

If you eat something too sugary, drink a couple of glasses of water, go for a brisk walk, find a dance floor and do your thing, drink some more and dance some more until you feel better.

### The Travails of the Travel Trail

On a recent trip to the USA, we discovered that American manufacturers don't label their cans and packets in the same way that we do in the UK, so there's no way of knowing how much sugar is inside something. Use common sense.

Sugar-free drinks are available in the USA, but there aren't that many in Europe. Unfortunately, our wonderful, concentrated squashes that you add to water are a phenomenon that is unknown in many other countries.

### Third World Countries

The last time I went to India was about twenty years ago. I discovered that they produce their own soft drinks and these are very good indeed, but I don't remember seeing any sugar free ones. They may have a local form of diet cola by now. They certainly sold bottled water, so you could buy some fruit juice and put some of it into your water for a change. If you love your "cuppa" as much as I do, you will be delighted to know that tea in India is absolutely terrific and the milk is like ours, so this will be one of the nicest cuppas you ever drink.

Every nationality knows about diabetes. It's actually a bigger problem among black, Asian and Jewish people than it is among Europeans, so there are doctors everywhere who can help you, but you may not find the same medicines that you're used to, and sometimes, you're also up against a language barrier.

There are shamans, sangomas, inangas and witchdoctors in various countries who will definitely understand your problem, but their choice of muti (rhymes with footie) will be somewhat interesting and exotic. Don't experiment too much...

You may get an opportunity for a massage or to join a meditation group or go for energy healing. These are good ideas.

### Goods from Overseas

Look carefully at food that you buy in the UK that originated in third world countries, because the labelling can be poor. I recently bought a Jamaican loaf cake that didn't mention sugar in the ingredients on the outside of the pack, but the paperwork inside showed that sugar was the main ingredient.

## *Emigration*

Find out as much as you can about your destined country before committing yourself to living there. Sign up with a doctor or hospital in the locality before you settle. If you're a refugee, take copies of your prescriptions with you. Find a Médecins Sans Frontières doctor as soon as you can.

## *Food and Holidays*

Choose an area, a hotel or a cruise where there's a variety of food to choose from, preferably in the form of a buffet. Sure, you'll be tempted by some things that you shouldn't have and you may inadvertently take in sugar or other things that you shouldn't have, but a few slip-ups on holiday probably won't kill you, as long as the majority of your fare is good. Also, you're more active on holiday, so this will help balance out any mishaps.

You may be less able to fight off germs than non-diabetics are, so in less-developed countries, eat vegetarian foods and ensure that the veggies are cooked, rather than salads (i.e. raw food). Alternatively, buy fruit and salad items, wash them in bottled water, and make yourself a picnic.

# 31

# Helpful Ideas

*Fatigue ~ Sore Skin ~ Cold ~ Dry Mouth and Bad Breath ~ Thrush for Men ~ Thrush for Women ~ Cystitis ~ Infections ~ Other Things ~ Sexual Problems ~ A Rude Story ~ Driving ~ A Selection of Oddments ~ A Strange Tail*

*I don't drink these days;*
*I'm allergic to alcohol and narcotics - I break out in handcuffs.*
Robert Downey Junior

## *Fatigue*
~ Don't volunteer for anything.
~ Think of ways to reduce your workload and never pressure on yourself. A good motto is, "Work smarter, not harder".
~ Put your feet up and take a nap when you can.
~ Don't fill up your children's lives with "activities" or things that are supposed to "improve" them.
~ If you have a baby, take a nap when the baby does.
~ If you're older and can't cope with long hours of work and housework, take naps and work at night if that's when you feel lively.

## *Sore Skin*
~ Most diabetics stick their feet out of the bedclothes, and I've heard of people wrapping their feet in cling film at night.

~ The seams in tight clothes will rub you.

~ If you're a woman, it's natural to want to be fashionable and to wear sexy clothes, but when you come home put on something sloppy and comfortable that doesn't rub.

~ Clothes labels often scratch the skin, so cut them out.

### Cold

~ Wear layers of clothing rather than one big sweater.

~ Cover your extremities with hats, scarves, gloves and warm socks to keep from losing body heat.

~ If your workplace is cold, buy a small fan heater for yourself.

### Dry Mouth and Bad Breath

Drink water and suck a sugar free peppermint, or use an occasional breath spray thingy.

### Thrush for Men

Thrush is a fungal infection that thrives on sugar. I think there are pills that you can take for it, but you will have to ask the chemist about this. Use an anti-fungal cream. Keep athlete's foot under control, as this is a related fungal problem.

### Thrush for Women

Most women get thrush now and again, even without diabetes, but it's a classic early indicator of diabetes. Attacks like to come at bank holidays, when you're on holiday, over Christmas or at some other inconvenient time, so here are some self-help tips:

~ Keep Canesten cream, pessaries, pills or whatever works for you in your medicine cupboard, in a makeup bag in your desk or locker at work. Take them with you if you travel.

~ Fungus loves a warm fusty environment, so avoid tights and nylon knickers until the attack is over.

~ Don't use bath salts, bubble bath, soap, shower cream or "intimate" perfume on the area - just bathe with warm water. Avoid scented loo paper.

~ Dip a tampon into a pot of plain bio yoghurt and use it for an hour or so. It may sound like science fiction when you realise that the yoghurt will "eat" the thrush. It's best not to think about this too much!

~ If the area outside the vagina is sore, dab it gently with some olive oil on a bit of clean cotton wool.

Thrush may be transferable from one person to another if the other person is also pre-disposed to it. Partners are always happy to keep away from bodily invasion, so give the sex a rest for a bit until you are better.

Avoid beer, vodka, whisky, Chinese, Malay, Thai or Japanese foods or anything else that contains soy sauce. Avoid tofu, mushrooms and other fungi, as all these can cause candida, and therefore, thrush. Avoid wheat, too. Once you're better, re-introduce these foods gradually.

### Cystitis

Men can get cystitis but it's a predominantly female ailment. Most women get cystitis on occasion even when they are not diabetic. Cystitis is extremely painful and the fever that accompanies it makes you really ill. The accumulation of sugar in the urine encourages germs to set up home there.

~ If you're prone to cystitis, buy at least two packs of an over-the-counter remedy and keep the boxes in the medicine cupboard, and in your desk or locker at work. Always take them with you if you travel. There are various makes of remedy on the market, and most consist of a box containing six packets of powder that you take in water over a period of two days.

~ If you think you have a bout of cystitis on the way, start the remedy immediately. If it doesn't go after one treatment, keep going with another box of powders.

~ If you can't get to a chemist, put baking powder (bicarbonate of soda) into water and drink that. It tastes like wallpaper paste but it will help.

~ Drink lots of water.

~ Avoid fruit juice, tea, coffee and soft drinks, as they are all acidic.

~ Don't eat fruit or tomatoes, as these are acidic.

~ Rest and keep warm.

~ Avoid tights, and wear cotton knickers until the attack is well over.

~ Avoid bath salts or bubble bath.

~ You won't fancy sex at this time, because you will be too ill and in too much pain, but I also suggest that you avoid it for a few days afterwards to give your bladder a chance to recover.

## Infections

~ Treat toothache as an emergency and get to the dentist as soon as possible.

~ Give in to a cold, stay at home in the warmth and coddle yourself.

~ If you get a chest infection, you may need antibiotics.

~ If you are (or become) allergic to certain antibiotics, you must add this information to your bracelet / necklace and the note or card you carry in your wallet or purse. This is really important, whether you are diabetic or not - you just don't need someone giving you a shot of some antibiotic that reacts with your body especially if you are unconscious at the time.

~ At the slightest hint of foot troubles of any kind, go to your doctor, diabetes clinic or podiatrist.

~ Don't be casual about cuts and scrapes, especially on the fingers. Use antiseptic creams and plasters. Wear plastic gloves when doing wet or mucky jobs.

## *Other Things*

~ If you get a nagging headache, drink a glass of water and have something to eat if you've missed a meal. If none of that helps, take headache pills.

~ If you get a zit just before an important date, bung some antiseptic cream on it and swear at it. Swearing won't make the zit go away, but it will make you feel better! Some people recommend putting a dab of toothpaste on zits before going to bed as that dries them out.

~ If your hair gets thin or falls out, consult a good hairdresser.

~ If you're irritable, go for a walk or do something sporty. Put some music on, then sing and dance around to it.

## *Sexual Problems*

I'm no sexpert, but there's help around for men whose erections aren't erecting properly. Your doctor may not ask you about your sex life, so you may need to raise the subject yourself. Nurses and doctors of both sexes hear this stuff all the time, so don't be embarrassed about speaking up. Some of your difficulties may be due to being unwell and things may improve once your diabetes and your general health improves. Some may be due to cholesterol problems, in which case improving your general health and lowering the cholesterol will do the trick. Some drugs (not necessarily for diabetes) can have an unfortunate effect. Much depends upon your age, as the male equipment doesn't work as well for anyone as they get older. The main thing is to tell your partner what's going on, so that she doesn't think you've gone off her or suspect that you've got someone else on the side.

You might be able to take Viagra or something similar, but you must ask your doctor about this. Don't be shy; he or she's heard it all many times before. Many years ago, a diabetic friend told me that he used a kind of bracelet thingy that wrapped around the base of his penis and testicles to make the penis hard. Maybe investigate the 'Net and perhaps visit an "adult" shop, as they must surely have heard just about everything related to these problems - and their solutions.

Don't drink too much, as that can affect any man's performance at any age, whether you're diabetic or in the best of health. Don't expect to be a great Don Juan if you're worried sick. Tackle the problems, lower the stress level and see how things improve.

Women can get vaginal dryness due to diabetes, getting older or both, so they will need a lubricant. Some lubricants damage condoms, so if your partner uses condoms, it is wise to ask your health care expert which type of product you should use. Avoid infections by washing the area before lovemaking and by having a pee afterwards, as this will wash out the urethra (the passage from the bladder). After sex, give the area a good wash. Tell the boyfriend to take his time, so that you can wallow in the sensations rather than trying to chase after an orgasm. I always think that an orgasm is like a feather; the more you chase it, the more it floats away from you. Buy a book on tantric sex!

## A Rude Story

If you don't like rude stories, don't read the next paragraph. This is an absolutely true story. It's a tale is about age rather than about diabetes, but you'll soon see why I've included it.

Years ago, we had a neighbour who was a bit of a joker. He told us that he sometimes used a certain London pub that was run by an "old guy". As it happened, the old chap had recently married a lady who was also getting on in years, and now they were back from their honeymoon. Our cheeky neighbour leaned over the bar and quietly asked the landlord, "I don't suppose you… well, you know what I mean?" The old boy looked him straight in the eyes and said, "Of course we did. Many times in fact! It was a bit like getting a marshmallow into a money-box, but we managed it!"

## Driving

You can drive a car, but you should keep some kind of notification about your diabetes in the car. In case of hypos, keep glucose sweets, biscuits and small cans of ordinary (i.e.

sugared) cola in the car. Also, keep small bottles of water in the car in case you get thirsty. If you're going through a bad patch, try to avoid very long and tiring journeys or trips in heavy traffic areas. Check your blood sugar before any potentially difficult journey, and if you feel lousy while travelling, stop the car and take a break, take a break and check your blood sugar. Perhaps you could keep a blood test kit in a small cool bag in the car for this purpose.

## *A Selection of Oddments*

~ Health and life insurance companies tend to welcome diabetics, because they take more care of themselves than other people do.

~ Any illness is expensive, but you will get your prescriptions free in the UK. If you eat properly, you may spend less on snacks, takeaways and junk food than others do.

~ There's no need to join an expensive gym or golf club, as the local leisure centre usually has some facilities.

~ Apparently a good sleeping pattern helps the insulin situation.

~ Tests show that those who snore are more likely to get diabetes than those who don't! Frankly, I'm not convinced about this one.

~ Some doctors say that all diabetics and pre-diabetics should be on statins to prevent heart disease or strokes. Others say that a healthy lifestyle is better.

## *A Strange Tail*

I've read that a diabetic's pet dog can detect an oncoming hypo and warn the diabetic in advance. Maybe these dogs have some special training for this, because all our dog can detect is din-dins, walkies or a bone!

# 32

# Supplements and Natural Remedies

---

*Natural Remedies ~ Treatments ~ Supplements ~ Meditation ~ Snake Oil ~ Astrology*

*One of the first duties of the physician is to educate the masses not to take medicine.*
Sir William Osler

### Natural Remedies

Natural remedies may help, but they won't take the place of proper treatment or of a proper eating and exercise regime. Never take anything in large quantities, as everything has side effects, and many so-called natural things are toxic in large quantities. Never take more than one or two things at one time, use one product for a couple of weeks and see if that makes any difference, then try something else. Only ever use a very little of anything. I can't guarantee the following listed results, as I haven't personally tried all these things:

~ Cinnamon to improve the introduction of insulin into the cells and reduce fats in the blood.

~ Nutmeg, for the same reasons as above.

~ Fenugreek to improve uptake of insulin into the cells.

~ Salacia oblonga to reduce blood sugar.

~ Garlic to lower blood fats (and keep away vampires...).

~ Ginkgo biloba for diabetic neuropathy (nerve damage).

~ Evening primrose for diabetic neuropathy (nerve damage).

~ Ginkgo biloba for memory. Diabetics need a good memory to take pills, take tests and remember what they ate last and when.

~ Dandelion root tea to help prevent heart and eye problems and it can help to normalise blood glucose.

~ Vitamin C in sizeable doses (up to 1,000 mg per day) does help the body to recover faster from damage, e.g. cuts, bruises, a cold and many other kinds of damage.

*Caffeine and guarana, which contains caffeine, were once considered helpful, but modern tests have shown that caffeine makes diabetes worse.*

### Treatments

Just off the top of my head, I can think of the following complementary therapies, but there are many others:

~ Acupuncture
~ Aromatherapy
~ Bach Flower Remedies
~ Neal's Yard Remedies
~ Shiatsu
~ Herbalism
~ Reflexology
~ Homeopathy

~ Reiki
~ Spiritual Healing
~ Naturopathy
~ Nutritional Therapy
~ Crystal Therapy
~ Zero Balancing
~ Osteopathy
~ Chiropractic
~ Geopathic Stress
~ Magnet therapy

One of the benefits of complementary practitioners is that they give their patients more time than an NHS doctor can, but some of their treatments might not fit with diabetes. It's probably best to avoid those that put things into the body, such as herbs, Bach Flower Remedies, Neal's Yard remedies and aromatherapy, because here the essential oils get in through the skin. Acupuncture and reflexology are said to be good for diabetes. Some reflexologists are too rough for easily damaged diabetic feet, so choose one who is known to be gentle.

Nutritional advice is very good and naturopathy might help, while massage and zero balancing also stimulate the body's ability to heal itself. The same goes for Reiki healing and spiritual or energy healing.

Geopathic stress treats the home and office, in a somewhat similar way to Feng Shui, but it is aimed at improving health.

Therapies and treatments must be complementary, which means that they complement or sit alongside conventional medicine, rather than taking its place.

These days, doctors are neither surprised nor put out by patients who use complementary therapies, so don't forget to tell your doctor about your therapy and your therapist about your medicines. They need to know, so they don't double up on treatments.

## Supplements

You might want to take one multivitamin a day and an extra dose of vitamin C if you have a cold or if you cut or damage yourself.

A multivitamin a day during winter is also a great way to stay healthy, even if you eat well. Just check the instructions, and don't double dose with other supplements at the same time. About the only thing that isn't a problem when overdosing, is Vitamin C, as the body doesn't keep it in the system for long.

Chromium is sometimes touted as an aid to diabetics and possibly even some kind of cure, but it isn't - in fact, chromium supplements aren't good for diabetics. It was tested on a group of malnourished Chinese peasants, and their diabetes improved - as did their general health - only once they had enough to eat. We eat many foods that contain trace elements such as chromium in our normal diet, so we normally don't need such additives, and metals can accumulate in the liver and organs.

## Meditation

You can contact Nina Ashby at the Foundation for Holistic Consciousness for her CDs and her book, Develop Your ESP published by Zambezi Publishing Ltd. When released, you may wish to try "Simply Meditation" - also published by Zambezi Publishing Ltd. Then, look on the Internet for other resources.

## Snake Oil

I get very irate at the people who sell rubbish to those who are vulnerable, or even those who are neurotic or easily taken in. If a bottle of green gunk can cure cancer, diabetes, sexual dysfunction, eczema and baldness, wouldn't the medical world have heard of it and adopted it for general use?

I remember an incident that happened when we took a stand at the annual Festival of Mind, Body & Spirit so that we could sell our books. Most of the people who work at these festivals are very honest, but as in all walks of life, there is a small minority who aren't. The trouble started when some freeloader asked us if we wouldn't mind putting a few leaflets on our table for them. Jan was new to the scene at the time, and he has a kind heart so he let the "shnorrer" do this. Soon, we had all kinds of leaflets being dumped onto our stand. I was in the process of collecting these up and shoving them in our rubbish bag, when a man came up and started talking to Jan. The guy was neatly dressed in a conventional shirt and tie and grey slacks, and he looked like a bog-standard office manager. He gave Jan a few small bottles of stuff and asked if he could put them on the stand. When we looked at the labels we could see that each bottle was supposed to cure something different, but when we studied the ingredients, we discovered that they were all the same, e.g. water and a few drops of grape alcohol. I threw the bottles away.

## Astrology

If you consult an astrologer, it can be a life enhancing experience. It may also show how you can improve your circumstances and work to make yourself happier.

If you're an astrologer yourself, look for the following possible indicators for diabetes, listed in order of importance:

~ Venus conjunct, opposite, square or semi-square to Saturn and/or Jupiter.

~ Mercury conjunct, opposite, square or semi-square to Saturn and/or Jupiter.

~ Afflictions to the sun. This is due to its rulership of the person as a whole, along with its connection to the "prana" or life force. In the chakra system, the sun rules the solar plexus chakra and the central areas of the body that are so involved with diabetes. These include the pancreas, liver and kidneys.

~ Look at planets in Virgo for digestion problems, including diabetes.

~ Planets in Libra for over-indulgence with food and alcohol, plus kidney problems.

~ Planets in Pisces for alcohol and foot problems.

~ Planets in Aries for alcohol and eye problems.

~ Planets in Scorpio for eye problems.

Sun signs alone don't shed much light on the subject, as diabetes seems to cross all the sun signs. Interestingly, Sister Yvonne Aitken says that diabetes is different from other conditions because it affects so much of the body and so many aspects of life. This parallels astrological theory, because every part of the body is involved. By this reasoning, diabetes may be inclined to have more effect on certain body parts, by sun sign connection, along the following lines:

| ZODIAC SIGN | BODY PART |
| --- | --- |
| Aries | eyes, brain and upper teeth |
| Taurus | lower teeth, throat infections |
| Gemini | chest infections, cuts on the hands |
| Cancer | pancreas, digestion |
| Leo | heart |
| Virgo | bowels |
| Libra | kidneys, bladder |
| Scorpio | genitals |
| Sagittarius | liver |
| Capricorn | shins |
| Aquarius | ankles, upper feet |
| Pisces | feet, toes |

# Conclusion

*Every cloud has a silver lining*

An old saying

### Conclusion

While researching this book, I learned that the methods of controlling diabetes from only a couple of decades ago no longer apply. Doctors now advocate a healthy eating regime that reduces sugars and fats and increases fibre, along with exercise, although many diabetics themselves still say they do better when on a lowish carbohydrate regime.

Do I do everything right myself? Not always. I get days when I eat sandwiches instead of meals, and there are days when I would rather watch telly than go out and exercise. For the most part I do the right thing, but age is catching up with me and my energy levels are not the same as they used to be.

Finally, if this book has confirmed to you that you are already doing all the right things, that's a very positive outcome. If you've learned things here that help you to improve your quality of life, and if this book helps just one person to avoid unnecessary problems, I will be really delighted.

**NB:** If you are a diabetic, please ask your loved ones to read this book, so that they can also start to understand this confusing ailment and the way it affects you.

Good luck from Sasha

# Bibliography

*Be careful of reading health books. You may die of a misprint.*
Mark Twain (1835 - 1910)

You are welcome to contact us with questions to do with Diabetes or other titles in our catalogue.

**Zambezi Publishing Ltd**
P.O. Box 221, Plymouth, PL2 2YJ
UK
Website: www.zampub.com
Email: info@zampub.com
*(please include the word "Diabetes" in the subject heading, to help distinguish your message from the tons of spam that we wade through).*
Phone: +44 (0) 1752 367 300
Fax:     +44 (0) 1752 350 453

***

**End the Food Confusion**
By Sonia Jones ND
Zambezi Publishing Ltd
Price: £12.99
This book is not specifically for diabetics; it's about good nutrition as a whole, including vitamins, digestion and health matters relating to food. Most of the advice and most of the recipes are absolutely fine for diabetics, but as with any other

book, you must look carefully at the contents of any recipe in the light of your own particular health needs.

**Quick Cooking for Diabetics**
In association with Diabetes UK
By Louise Blair and Norma McGough
Hamlyn
£5.99

**The New Diabetic Cookbook**
By Mabel Cavaini
McGraw Hill
£8.99

**Complete Cookery Diabetic**
By Jacqueline Bellefontaine
Silverdale Books
£14.99
(This book may not be readily available. Try giving Bookmart a call, as they own Silverdale and they may have stocks. Also try Amazon or Abe Books, as they may have a cheapo or even a second hand copy).

**Diabetic Cookbook**
By Paul Morgan
Bookmart Ltd
Quantum Publishing Ltd
Price: £9.99
(This is like the one above. Try Bookmart, Amazon or Abe Books online.)

**The Diabetes Weight Loss Diet**
In association with Diabetes UK
By Anthony Worrall Thompson, Azmina Govindji, Jane Suthering
Kyle Cathie Ltd
Price: £12.99

**GI & GL Counter**
By Dr Wynnie Chan
Published by Hamlyn, a division of Octopus Publishing Group Ltd
Price: £7.99
This explains the GI and GL indices and shows which are high, medium and low by numbers and by an easy key.

**The South Beach Diet**
By Dr Arthur Agatston
Rodale Ltd
Price: £4.99
This lists a huge variety of foods by their carbohydrates, fats, calories and so on. It also tells you which to avoid, and which to eat some of or lots of. It's not specifically for diabetics, but for those who want to lose weight. As carbohydrates are a major problem for many diabetics, the information in this book could be useful.

**The Reverse Diabetes Diet**
By Dr Neal D Bernard
Rodale
£12.99
This book advocates a vegan diet.

**Healthy Eating for Diabetes**
By Antony Worrall Thompson and Azmina Govindji
(I saw this on the 'Net and I don't have a copy myself, so I don't have any more info on it).

*Books about Diabetes*

**Diabetes for Dummies**
By Dr Sarah Jarvis, GP & Alan L Rubin, MD
Published by John Wiley & Sons Ltd
I couldn't find a price for this one.
Make sure that you get the UK edition, or the blood test measurements and several other things won't make sense. This is an excellent and very comprehensive book.

**Type 2 Diabetes, Your Questions Answered**
By Rosemary Walker & Jill Rogers
Dorling Kindersley
£9.99
This is good, basic book that answers all those frequently asked questions.

**Type 2 Diabetes**
CSF Medical Communications Ltd.
£5.99
This gives excellent information about the medicines that diabetics take, among other things.

**The Diabetes Guide**
Written by NHS diabetes professionals, edited by Adam Daykin
Virgin Books Ltd
Price: £10.99

**Living With Type 2 Diabetes**
Gloria Loring and Dr Timothy J Gray DO
M Press, 10956 SE Main Street, Milwaukee, OR 97222
Despite its title, much of this book is suitable for type 1 diabetics as well as type 2 diabetics who have to deal with medication or insulin injections. This is easy to read and it is useful for all diabetics, but especially for those whose diabetes is fairly severe.

**Diabetes - the Complete Guide**
By Dr Rowan Hillson
Random House Ltd
Price: £9.99
This is very thorough and it takes things much further than my book does, so it is suitable for those whose diabetes is at any level, from mild to severe.

**The First Year: Type 2 Diabetes**
By Gretchen Becker
Robinson
£9.99
This is similar in style to my book, partly because the author is a writer rather than a doctor or nurse. She is also a diabetic, so she writes from the standpoint of day-to-day reality rather than scientific theory, and she obviously has a great deal of common sense. This book is worth reading as a follow up to mine, because it goes into scientific detail about treatments, etc.

**Type 2 Diabetes, Your Questions Answered**
By Rosemary Walker & Jill Rodgers
Dorling Kindersley
Price: £9.99

**A Simple Guide to Type 2 Diabetes**
By various authors
DSF Medical Communications Ltd.
Price: £5.99

**Outsmart Diabetes**
Edited by Dawn Bates (no single author)
Rodale
£9.99
This is a very basic introduction to diabetes.

**Diabetes UK**

I repeat the information here from the introductory part of this book.

"Balance" is a wonderful magazine produced for diabetics. It's sometimes available in shops like W H Smith, but it's published by Diabetes UK.

If you would like to become a member of Diabetes UK, call free on 0800 138 5605 or visit www.diabetes.org.uk/jointoday

For further information, call the Customer Services team on 0845 123 2399 during office hours.

Diabetes UK

10 Parkway

London NW1 7AA

www.diabetes.org.uk/balance

Telephone: 020 7424 1000

Diabetes UK offers a membership scheme to help people attain good management of their diabetes. It keeps members up to date with diabetes developments and connects them to a network of people who understand the condition.

Diabetes UK also posts useful information on its website.

## *Useful Websites*

www.glycaemicindex.com

www.mendoza.com/diabetes.htm

www.moodfoodcompany.co.uk

www.tescoDiets.com/diabetes

**The Diabetes Monitor**

*Resource for patients to educate themselves about their role as active participants in care of their condition.*

www.diabetesmonitor.com

**International Diabetic Athletes Association**

For diabetes and sport

www.diabetes-exercise.org

**NHS Direct**
24-hour helpline. Includes a section on diabetes.
www.nhsdirect.nhs.uk

*Magazines for Healthy Lifestyles and Nutrition*
Brand New You
Celebrity Diet Now
Easy Living
Eating for Your Health
Fresh
Good Food
Health & Fitness
Here's Health
In Balance Health & Lifestyle Magazine
Journal of Alternative & Complementary Medicine
Lighter Life
Men's Health
Natural Health
Organic Life
Sainsbury's Magazine
Slim at Home
Slimmer, Healthier, Fitter
Slimming Magazine
Spa World
Therapy Weekly
Top Santé Health & Beauty
The Vegan Society
Weight Watchers Magazine
Women's Fitness
Women's Health
Yoga and Health
Your Essential Lifescape
Zest

# Index

**A**

A&E 9
acesulfame 60
acetone 41
Activity 95
aerobics 97
Afro-Caribbean 16
agave nectar 106
age 74
Aitken, Sister Yvonne 4, 13, 184
alcohol 42, 43, 55, 56, 123, 141, 158, 159, 162, 167
Alcoholics Anonymous 56
Alcopop 142
allergies 159
almonds 23
Alternatives 54
Alzheimer's 42
amputation 5
amputations 14
ankles 42
antibiotics 135, 174
apples 61
Apprentice, The 68
apricots, dried 64

aromatherapy 54
arrogance 9
arteries 64
arteries, hardening of the 14
arthritis 23
Ashby, Nina 182
Asian, South East 16
aspartame 60
astrology 183
athlete's foot 41, 156, 172
A-type 68
A-type, wannabe 68
autoimmune reaction 34
Avocados 64
Avoid 143

**B**

baby 77
baby-boomers 16
Bacon 101, 105, 123
bagels, brown 101
baking 60
baking powder 174
bananas 139
bath salts 173, 174
Beans 76, 83, 131, 132, 140

beans, red kidney 131
beef 122
Beef burgers 66
beer 143
beer, ginger 144
beta cells 14, 34, 80
bicarbonate of soda 152, 174
Biscuits 107
BlackBerry 68
bladder 152, 174
blindness 5, 14, 150
blindness, temporary 40
blister 97
blisters 41
blood glucose 23, 50, 145
blood pressure 14, 50, 75, 151
blood test 48
blood test machine 92
BMI 71, 74
Body Mass Index 71
bones, crumbling 14
bracelet 26, 43, 161, 174
bracelet, magnetic 55
bracelets 27, 95
bread, banana 106
bread, granary 64, 83, 118
bread, pita 109
bread, white 109, 126
bread, wholegrain 140
Breads 127
breakfast 83
Breakfast, Continental 101
breastfeeding 77
breath, fresh 153
Brie 66, 110
buck 65

buckwheat 21
Buffets 117
burger 121
burning 153
butter 66, 76, 137
butter, spread-able 66

**C**

caduceus 27
Caffeine 101, 147, 180
cake, high fibre 84
cakes 107
CALORIES 145
cancer, bowel 140
cancer, breast 5
Canderel 60, 61
candida 23, 122, 173
carbohydrate 121, 131
carbohydrates 22, 43, 57, 63, 136
carbohydrates, high fibre 63
Carbohydrates, useful 125
cards, laminated 161
care, every-day 154
careers 25
Caroline 46
carrots 105
Carvery 119
casserole 133
cassoulet 133
cataracts 40
Causes 16
celery 110
cereal 152
cereal bars 111
Cereals 100

chakra system 54
Checklist 18
Cheddar 66
Cheese 66, 110, 136
cheese, cottage 136
chemicals 135
chicken 122, 133
chicken Kiev 126
chicken, barbeque 123
chicken, cooked 123
chicken, Fried 121
chips 67
chiropodist 155
chocolate 58, 111, 114
chocolate, hot 147
choices, good 127
choices, poor 127
choleric personality 68
cholesterol 22, 23, 42, 50, 56,
63, 65, 75, 76, 104, 109, 121,
137, 151, 175
cholesterol, bad 64
cholesterol, Good 64
cholesterol, Total 50
Christmas 157
chromium 182
cider 142
Cigareeets and Whisky 55
cinnamon 84, 180
Cocktail Ideas 146
cocoa powder 136
cocoa, black 147
coffee 124, 147
coffee, Decaffeinated 147
coffee, Latte 147
cold 151, 172

colds 19
coleslaw 121
colours, different 139
coma 43, 53
complementary therapies 54
conditioners 156
conjunctivitis 150
constipation 152
contact lenses 150
cooking 60
cornstarch 21, 111
cough medicines 156
countries, Third World 168
couscous 110, 126
cream 76, 137, 158
cream, antiseptic 175
crudités 105
Crumpets 101
crusts 41
crystal healing 55
currants 111
curry 105
custard, sugar-free 106, 137
cuts 18, 41, 150, 151, 174
cystitis 19, 41, 146, 152, 173

**D**
Dairy 136
dancing 152
dancing, salsa 97
dancing, tap 97
Dandelion root 180
dates 111, 140
DBML 162
dehydration 41, 152
dentist 64

dextrose 123
Diabetes 6, 13, 163
diabetes mellitus 39
Diabetes UK 4, 5, 78, 87, 92
diabetes, borderline 31, 32
Diabetes, Childhood type 2 33
diabetes, Diet-controlled 32
diabetes, Gestational 78
diabetes, mature onset 33
diabetes, Mild 32
Diabetes, Non-Severe Type 2 97
diabetes, type 1 14, 34, 92, 96
Diabetes, Type 1.5 33
diabetes, type 2 14, 33, 92
diabetes, undiagnosed 31
Diabetes, Varieties of 32
diabetic children 87
diabetic parents 89
Diabetic Products 60, 114
Diabetics, Famous 26
diarrhoea 60, 61, 153
Diet 21
diet, healthy 63
diet, high fat 63
diet-control 97
Dinner Parties 117
Disposal 47
DIY 151
dogs 17, 177
donkey 65
Dragon's Den 68
drinks, herbal 147
drinks, no-added-sugar 146
drinks, sugar free soft 167
drinks, sugar-free 168
driving 176
DVLA 26, 53

**E**
Edam 66, 110
egg, scrambled 67
eggs 67, 76, 109, 153
emigration 169
emotions 42
erection, full 41
espresso 147
Ethnicity 16
Evening primrose 180
exchanges 57
exercise 14, 43, 79
experts 9
extremities 172
eye test 15, 28
eyes 56, 149
eyesight 18

**F**
fasting 49
fat, excess 21
fat, hydrogenated 64, 76
fat, saturated 21
Fatigue 40, 171
Fats 50, 63, 64, 135
fats, homogenised 64
feet 14, 41, 42, 153
Fenugreek 180
fibre 105, 139
figs 111, 140
first aid 53

fish 66, 67, 76, 104, 118, 121, 135, 136
fish, Oily 136
flour, white 21, 23, 111
food poisoning 41
food, buffet 157
food, canned 104
food, dairy 66
food, deli 136
food, fatty 67
food, fried 67
food, Italian 122
food, low GI 70
food, normal 21
food, organic 59
food, processed 79
food, shortages of 16
food, Starchy 104
foods, Deli 65
footwear, special 166
formalin 60
fruit 22, 63, 77, 106, 139, 174
fruit salad 117
fruit, Canned 106
fruit, citrus 152
fruit, dried 140
fruits, tropical 126
full fat 6
fungal infection 172

**G**
gardening 6
Garlic 180
geopathic stress 181
ghee 76, 119
GI 69, 126, 139

GI, high 69
GI, low 69
gin 143
Ginkgo biloba 180
glaucoma 40
glucose 6, 14
glucose sweets 43
glucose tablets 96
glucose tolerance test 49
gluten-free 137
Glycaemic Index 69, 126
goji beans 21
Gouda 66, 110
Grapefruit 101
grapes 139
Gravy 103
grilling 82
grit 165
grouse 65
guarana 180

**H**
H45 cream 41
hair 156
Halal 123
ham 122
hands 151
Hawking, Stephen 13
HbA1c 49, 50
headache 175
Headaches 41
heart 151
heart attack 42
heart attacks 14, 68
heart disease 56, 177
herbal medicine 54

Hermes 27
high blood pressure 64
holiday 61, 164
Holidays, Feet and 164
homeopathy 54
hormones, endomorphic 95
hospital, St Mary's 143
hydrogenated oil 137
hypo 43, 53, 78, 96, 145, 177
hypo pickup 111
hypo, nocturnal 88
Hypoglycaemia 43, 123, 145
hypoglycaemic 25, 42, 56, 92
hypos 176
hysterectomy 74

**I**
icecream 106
icecream, diabetic 137
icecream, low calory 137
ID Cards 27
ignorance 9
Impaired fasting glycaemia 32
Impaired glucose tolerance 32
impulse buying 82
inangas 168
infection 41, 153
infections 150, 174, 176
insects, stinging 166
insulin 6, 14, 26, 33, 56, 78,
80, 92, 97, 163
insulin, Inhalant 34
insurance, holiday 26
insurance, life 177
insurers, motor 26

**J**
Jewish disease 16
jobs 25
juice, fruit 106
juice, Pure fruit 147
juice, tomato 123

**K**
Karen 158
karma 17
kebab 120
ketchup 58
ketoacidosis 41
kidney damage 40
kidney dialysis 14
kidneys 14, 42
kippers 101
Kosher 123

**L**
labelling 59, 137, 168
lactic acid 136
lager 142
languages, other 162
lard 64, 76
lasagna 105
Lauren 46
legs 14
lentils 131
liposuction 83
liver 14, 56, 80, 92
lobster 66
lubricants 176
lunch snack 111
lunch, packed 109
Lynne 29

**M**

mackerel 66
marshmallow 176
Martini, Dry 143
massage 55, 181
mayonnaise 59, 105
meals on wheels 123
Meals, Skipping 80
Measurements 46
measurements, Liquid 55
meat 64, 131, 135
MedicAlert 26, 27, 43, 161
medication 26, 53
medication, essential 163
medication, prescribed 28
medicine, conventional 181
Melon 106
melons 126, 139
Mercury 27
metabolism 74
mg/dl 51
migraine 40
milk 11, 66, 136
milk puddings 22
milk, semi-skimmed 66, 76
milk, skimmed 76
minerals 120, 126
Misconception 31
mixers 144
money-box 176
muscles 14
mushrooms 23, 67, 173
mustards 109
muti 168

**N**

nap 171
National Health Service 92
naturopathy 181
necklace 26, 27, 95, 174
nerve damage 56
nerve endings 97, 153
nerve pains 42
neuropathy 180
Neurosis 47
NHS 10
Noodles 133
Nutmeg 180
nuts 64, 83, 111

**O**

Obesity 5, 33, 71
oil, olive 64, 67, 76
oil, rapeseed 64
oil, sunflower 64, 67
oil, vegetable 23
ointment 165
omega 3 66, 104
omega 6 104
Ostrich 65
ovaries, Polycystic 41
overweight 15, 75
overweight teenagers 81

**P**

pain 42
pain, stabbing 153
pancreas 14, 33, 78, 92
Parkinson's 42
parsnips 105, 126, 139
partridge 65

pasta 110
pasta, brown 23
pasta, wholegrain 140
pasties 65, 111
Pâté 65, 76, 119
peanut butter 64
Pearson, Nurse Sue 3
peas 131, 140
penicillin 154
people, nasty 89
pepperoni 65
pessaries 172
pets 17
Pharmacists 93
pickles 58
Pies 65, 111
pies, mince 158
pillbox 92
pills 43, 56, 97, 172
Pills, Contraceptive 77
pills, glucose 78
Pilsner 143
pizza 105, 122
placenta 78
plasters 165
ploughman's lunch 122
polyps 140
popcorn 126, 129
porridge 99, 140
potassium chloride 75
Potato crisps 114
potato, baked 70
potatoes 83, 153
potatoes, new 105, 125
potatoes, old 121, 126
potatoes, sweet 105, 125

Poultry 65, 118, 135, 136
practitioners, complementary 181
prawns 66, 121
Pre-diabetes 32, 74
Pre-diabetic 91
pregnancy 16, 77
prescriptions 177
prescriptions, free 93
protein 121, 131, 136
prunes 152
pub grub 121
pudding, Milk 106
purse 26

Q
quinoa seeds 21

R
ratatouille 67
recipe 132
recipes 22, 23
reflexology 55
remedies, natural 179
Restaurants 118
retinopathy 40, 42, 150
rice 22, 83, 106
rice, Basmati 104, 126
rice, boiled 76, 119
rice, brown 23, 126
rice, long grain 126
rolls 122
rolls, brown 122
roughage 140

**S**

sago 106
Salacia oblonga 180
salad dressings 58, 59
salad, Russian 110
salads 76, 83, 105, 139
salami 65, 76, 135
salami factory 65
salmon 109
salsa dancing 6
salt 21, 111, 135, 136, 151
salt, common table 75
Salt, Lo 75
sandals 155, 164, 166
Sandwiches 122
sangomas 168
sardines 66
Sasha's Cake Recipe 85
sauce, cranberry 158
sauce, soy 173
sauces 58
sausage rolls 111
sausage, liver 65
sausages 64, 105, 135, 136
school 87
schoolchildren 140
scrapes 151, 174
seeds 64
self-help 4
semolina 22, 106
sensitivity 150
sex life 175
shamans 168
shampoos 156
Shape 74
shellfish 103, 104

sherry 143
shins 42
Shiraz 143
shock 29, 30
Shoes 97, 154
shoes, buying 165
shopping list 80, 82
shrimps 66
Singapore 163
siphon 39
skin 18, 40, 150
skin cancer 42
skin, broken 151
skin, sore 172
sleep 18
slimming 79
Slimming World 80
slippers 154
Smoking 55, 74
smoothies 139
snacks 111
socks 155
Sodit 80
sodium 23
Sodium chloride 75
solar keratosis 42
soup 83, 103, 105, 111, 132
soups, packet 131
soya 23
Spikes 53
spirits 142, 143
spiritual healing 55
Splenda 22, 60, 61, 106, 136
sports 25, 48
sports, extreme 97
spreads 22, 66

spritzer 143
stamina 84
starch 131
statins 177
stew 133
sties 150
stillbirth 78
stir-fry 67
stomach bands 83
stomach upset 61
strawberries 119, 158
stress 13, 29, 40, 157, 167
Stress Levels 54
stroke 42
strokes 14, 68, 177
sucralose 60
sugar content 140
sugar, fruit 22, 61, 106
Sugars 128
sugars, natural 139
sunlight 11
suntan cream 165
supplements 182
surgery 83
Survivors 82
Swedes 105, 126, 139
sweet foods 58
sweetcorn 140
sweeteners 22, 60, 124, 128
sweets 21
Symptoms 36, 39
syringes 164

**T**
tai chi 97, 98
takeaways 76

Tale of Three Croissants 54
tandoori 76
tannin 148
tapas 123
tapioca 22, 106
tea 118, 124, 147
tea, rooibos 147
teachers 88
teens 88
teeth 19, 153
Tesco 80
therapies, complementary 180
thirsty 18
thrush 19, 41, 122, 172, 173
tikka 76
tingling 40, 153
tingling feelings 18
toes 14
tofu 173
tomato juice 162
tomatoes 110, 174
tooth decay. 41
toothache 174
tortilla 109
trace elements 139
trans fats 64, 76, 137
treacle 140
Triglyceride level 50
triglycerides 56, 63
Trinity 88
tummy bug 164
tummy bugs 19
Tuna 109
turkey 65

**U**
ulcer 42
ulcers 159
urine strip 45
UV light 166

**V**
veganism 23
vegetable oils 64
vegetables 63, 77, 83, 105, 139
veins 64
verruca 156
Viagra 175
vinegar 104
vision 40, 53, 149
vitamin C 180
vitamin D 10
vitamin supplements 156
vitamins 126, 139
vodka 143
vomiting 41

**W**
Waist measurement 50
Waist size 71
wallet 26
war babies 16
wart remover 156
wartime rationing 16
water 120, 123, 140, 146, 158, 162, 167, 174
weather, hot 167
weight 18
Weight Watchers 106, 143, 158

weight, apple-shaped 74
weight, excess 79
weight, losing 80
weight, Pear-shaped 74
weird 96
wheat 173
wheat, bulgur 126
wheat, durum 110
whisky 143
Wild, Wild Women 56
wine, red 143
wine, white 142
witchdoctors 168

**Y**
yams 105, 125
yeast 122
yoghurt 101, 106

**Z**
zero balancing 181
zits 41

*Zambezi Publishing Ltd*

We hope you have enjoyed reading this book. The Zambezi range of books includes titles by top level, internationally acknowledged authors on fresh, thought-provoking viewpoints in your favourite subjects. A common thread with all our books is the easy accessibility of content; we have no sleep-inducing tomes, just down-to-earth, easily digestible, credible books.

~~~~~

Please visit our website at www.zampub.com to browse our full range of Lifestyle and Mind, Body & Spirit titles, and to see what might spark your interest next...

~~~~~

***Please note:-***

Our books are available from good bookshops throughout the UK, but nowadays, no bookshop can hope to carry in stock more than a fraction of the books published each year (over 200,000 new titles were published in the UK last year!). However, most UK bookshops can order and supply our titles swiftly, in no more than a few days (within the UK). If they say not, that's incorrect.

You can also find all our books on amazon.co.uk, other UK internet bookshops, and many are also on amazon.com; sometimes under different titles and ISBNs. Look for the author's name.

Our website (www.zampub.com) also carries and sells our whole range, direct to you. If you prefer not to use the Internet for book purchases, you are welcome to contact us direct (address is at the front of this book) for pricing and payment methods.

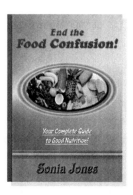

# End the Food Confusion

## Sonia Jones ND

Nutritional information is often confusing, contradictory, complicated and impractical. Sonia's book takes us through the values and contents of a huge variety of food and vitamins, to show clearly what actually happens to our bodies when we treat them well, or how we damage them by eating badly.

~~~~~

This book is for everyone, including vegetarians and dieters, with a terrific range of delicious recipes for most requirements. Sonia takes a sensible view of what comprises a balanced and healthy diet, thus allowing us to choose, easily and naturally, the right mix for a healthy, zest-filled lifestyle.

~~~~~

Sonia Jones is a qualified Naturopath, Dietary Therapist and Reflexologist, with years of experience in Australia, and running her own clinics in the UK and Malta.

She has now achieved her long-standing ambition of creating a first-class clinic in Valle Escondido, a beautiful spot in Panama, where she specialises in chronic illness and holistic diet programs, along with a variety of naturopathic therapies.

ISBN 978-1-903065-72-3     272 pages     RRP £12.99

Printed in the United Kingdom
by Lightning Source UK Ltd.
133674UK00001BB/94-279/P

9 781903 065686